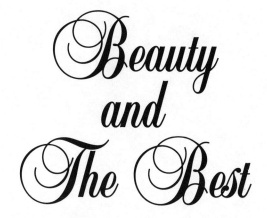

Beauty
and
The Best

Also by Debra Evans

The Complete Book on Childbirth

Heart & Home

Without Moral Limits

The Woman's Complete Guide to Personal Health Care

---

*If you are interested in having Debra Evans come speak to your
church or special event, please contact:*
interAct Speaker's Bureau
330 Franklin Road, Suite 120
Brentwood, TN 37024-0897
Voice: (615) 370-9937
Fax: (615) 370-9939

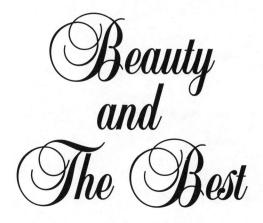

Beauty and The Best

Debra Evans

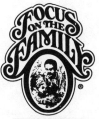

PUBLISHING
Colorado Springs, CO 80995

Library of Congress Cataloging-in-Publication Data
Evans, Debra.
Beauty / Debra Evans.
1st ed.
Includes bibliographical references and index.
ISBN 1-56179-178-4
1. Beauty—popular works. I. Title.

Published by Focus on the Family Publishing, Colorado Springs, Colorado 80995.
Distributed by Word Books, Dallas, Texas.

Editor: Gwen Weising
Cover Design: Margy Coleman for David Reilly & Associates

Printed in the United States of America
93 94 95 96 97 98/ 9 8 7 6 5 4 3 2 1

To my sisters,
Kerry and Nancy, with love

Table of Contents

Acknowledgments

Part One: The Diagnosis

Part Two: The Cure

Acknowledgments

In the fall of 1990, I received a letter from my friend Alice Lawhead, in which a clipping from the London *Sunday Times* was enclosed. I didn't realize it then, but the article she sent planted the seed that later grew into this book. Somehow, Alice knew that I'd find the topic to be as irresistible as her cooking. On both sides of the Atlantic, I've appreciated her company and timely hospitality tremendously, and am grateful for her unique ministry to Christian writers.

Jana Davila was a constant source of encouragement as we discussed research and statistics over the course of two years (and at least a dozen breakfasts!) at Le Peep.

Mike Hyatt, my former editor and publisher, also played an integral role in nurturing the book's concept. He also introduced me to St. John Chrysostom. Mike became my agent at a time when I was particularly discouraged due to several of my books going out of print. As the father of five daughters, Mike was *especially* enthusiastic about a book being written on the subject of beauty from a biblical perspective! Mike's partner, Robert Wolgemuth, was particularly helpful to my husband and me during initial stages of decision-making and as the publication date of the book grew closer. Their professionalism as business associates and innovative leaders in the area of author representation makes it a joy to work with them.

Special thanks also goes to those who endorsed the book early on: Susan Yates, Connie Marshner, Beverly LaHaye, and George Grant. Your willingness to read the manuscript on such short notice was greatly appreciated. To Sandy

VanderZicht, Scott Bolinder, Carol Johnson, Lavonne Neff, and Eileen Mason, I also extend my deep appreciation.

At Focus on the Family, there are a number of people I would like to thank—Rolf Zettersten, for giving the final go-ahead; Al Janssen, for his oversight of the book's publication and the warm welcome he extended to Dave and me on a chilly night in Chattanooga; Carol Ann Senger, for taking care of the details; Gwen Weising, my thoughtful editor and coach, for going past the call of duty to get everything wrapped up by the end of July; Megan Horne, for fine-tuning the manuscript and matching up endnotes by phone; Deb Nelson, for helping put the pieces together; Beverly Rykerd, for getting the publicity going on time and working with my freelance photographer, Judy Schlenker (thanks, Judy!), so efficiently; Nancy Wallace, for developing and implementing strategies that made the difference; and Dr. James Dobson, for his visionary leadership and a steady, loving commitment to Jesus that's an abiding example to us all. It's a privilege to work with you!

Barb Woodhead, Lori Marcuson, Carol Newsom, Laurel Justice, Linda King, Emmy Nelson, Shawn Lohry, Kim Citro, Janet Smith, Judith Markham, Kathy Nesper, Theresa Dalton, Pam Yaksich, and the board and staff at Bethany Christian Services in Atlanta—no words can adequately express my gratitude for your friendship, prayers, and timely ministrations.

Beyond this, I owe the successful completion of *Beauty and the Best* to my family: my husband, Dave; my children, Joanna, Katherine, David, Jonathan, and son-in-law, Matthew White; my parents, John and Nancy Munger; and my sisters, Kerry and Nancy. I thank God for the bonds we share, and for your continuing love, which you make real to me in remarkable ways when I need it most.

Part One

�֍❦֍

The Diagnosis

One

Captive To Beauty

What is beautiful is also good,
and who is good will soon be beautiful.
       —*Sappho,* Fragment, *c. 610 B.C.*

What we wish beauty to be is not
necessarily the same as what beauty is.
—*Arthur Marwick,* Beauty in History, *1988*

I work out and I can't eat anything and have to struggle all the time," Cindy Crawford, the 26-year-old beauty who holds multimillion dollar modeling contracts with Pepsi and Revlon, recently explained. She lamented: "I *still* feel insecure about the way I look." [1]

Supermodels Kim Alexis, Carol Alt, and Beverly Johnson recount similar feelings and experiences. In a joint interview, the three women—who between them have appeared on more than 2,000 magazine covers— spoke frankly about the stresses and health problems of struggling to stay at the peak in the beauty business.[2]

Alexis, who is five-feet-ten-inches tall, admits that after being discovered by a talent scout, the owner of New York City's Elite modeling agency guaranteed her "a certain amount of money" if she lost 15 pounds.[3] At the time, she weighed 145 pounds. "I cried for the first year of my career," Alexis confesses honestly. "I remember trying every fad diet. I remember starving myself for four days in a row. I remember trying the Atkins diet, which was low carbohydrate, high protein. If I didn't drop ten pounds in a week, I was on to another diet." As a result, Alexis points out, "I lost my period for a full two years." [4]

Carol Alt also dieted and exercised strenuously to force her five-foot-eight-inch frame down to an unnaturally slender 115 pounds. On her first modeling job, she passed out and fell into fellow model Kelly Emberg's arms. "An editor had given me a month to lose 12 pounds," Alt explains. "If I did, she promised me a trip to Rome for a shoot. I had never been to Rome. So I stopped eating." [5]

As a highly paid fashion model and cover girl, Beverly Johnson frequently found herself doing exactly the same thing. "I ate nothing. I mean *nothing*," she says. "From the moment I took my first picture, I thought it would be my last, and from the moment I started modeling at 17-years-old, I thought that the next 16-year-old girl who came in would be better than me." [6] Eventually ending up with bulimia, anorexia, and a thyroid problem, Beverly attributes her ailments to self-imposed starvation and crash dieting. "In our profession, clothes look better on a hanger, so you have to look like a hanger," Johnson points out. "It will never change." [7]

"It takes two hours to put on *natural* make-up," Alt observes pointedly. "Anybody who thinks that society pressures women to live up to our image should think of what we have to go through to maintain that image." [8]

Models aren't the only public images faced these days with the reality of constant whittling and shaping of their bodies. Actresses such as Demi Moore, Kathleen Turner and Linda Hamilton reportedly work out five to eight hours daily with personal trainers to achieve the "look" their directors want. In recent years, a steady succession of celebrities have revealed the results of their plastic surgeries on television talk shows and in popular magazines. The "look" being promoted on billboards and movie screens today, while increasingly unrealistic for women to obtain, is portrayed as a reasonable—even desirable—goal. Yet, as we view these images through the distorted lens of our image-conscious society, we wonder how we, too, can improve our appearance.

A Tale of Three Sisters

As the oldest of three daughters, I learned at an early age that it's preferable to be pretty because *looking good promotes success*—a belief that distorts the simple pleasures of one's femininity or finding enjoyment in the practice of good grooming.

Over the years this creed exacted its toll on my sisters and me in different ways. Eating disorders, failed friendships, work-related difficulties, rejection from others, cosmetic surgery, debt, sexual temptations, and depression are a few of the things we've encountered. Just as millions of women struggle today, including the famous models and actresses mentioned above, we were face-to-face with the unrealistic expectations of "beauty."

In the long run, my sisters and I have been affected in different ways by society's expectations concerning beauty. I experimented with clothes and cosmetics early and relished the pursuit before my sisters did. Growing up, I especially enjoyed getting ready for special occasions when I wore red velvet and lace, shiny black shoes, anklets with white ruffles, satin bows in my hair, and creamy smooth lip gloss. I'll always remember graduating from sixth grade when everything I wore, from head to toe, was brand new. I felt new, too.

Later, in seventh grade, I began wearing nylons and Capezios; and I put aqua-colored magnetic curlers the size of orange juice cans in my hair to curl it. In eighth grade, I used scotch tape to straighten my bangs, sticking the messy stuff across the front and sides of my by-then-super-short hair every night before going to bed. By ninth grade, applying mascara and blush had turned into a twice-a-day ritual; by tenth, I asked for a facial steamer, cologne, and a subscription to *Seventeen* for Christmas.

As the beauty cult of the sixties took off, I soared right along with it—including Mary Quant make-up and all. My junior year in high school, I worked every Saturday at a downtown Detroit boutique named "Hyperbole," owned by two of my favorite high school teachers. A tall, thin, green-eyed blonde with high cheekbones and a clear complexion, I bought clothes from the boutique and thoroughly enjoyed the extra attention I received because of the way I looked and the clothes I wore.

By the time I turned sixteen, I had already acquired a beg-borrow-or-steal mentality concerning clothing and cosmetics: I was ready and willing to do whatever it took to obtain the look I wanted. I once "borrowed" my mom's credit cards and charged about two hundred dollars' worth of makeup and expensive fabric without her permission, then sewed several of the shortest dresses I could design. I dieted constantly to keep my five-foot-eight-inch frame under 120 pounds, developing bulimia in the process. I tried to keep my legs lean, long, and continually on display. Even my wedding dress was "mini," with a thigh-length hem that barely reached my fingertips. It was fun for a while, but eventually, I ended up living out a kind of beauty that traps rather than transforms. Its power is real, and the myth that it teaches—that it's best to be beautiful because beauty *is* best—is a lie.

When I started following Christ in 1971, I abandoned costly cosmetics and skimpy clothes in favor of hand-sewn garments and blue jeans—not so much as a result of my newly found faith, but because I couldn't afford expensive fashion and beauty items. It was actually a relief not to play the glamour game any longer. Men no longer stared at me when I walked down the street, and I knew that my friends liked me for who I was, rather than for my appearance.

Today, I don't have a lot of money to invest in cosmetics and clothes, but I am confronted on a daily basis by decisions about clothing, cosmetics, and how to think about my body. The pressure to look good still remains because of the culture in which I live.

Watching my sisters' struggles, in this regard, illustrates that my own journey is far from unique. Kerry, who is four years my junior, is unable to gain weight due to intestinal surgery she had as a child. Consequently, she'll probably never be larger than a size four, and at five-foot-nine, her thinness is deemed a considerable accomplishment these days. In many people's minds, the Ph.D. that Kerry is earning in education from a top university pales in comparison to the amazing "achievement" of looking like a model.

My youngest sister Nancy, 10 years my junior, went to the same high school as rock star Madonna, graduating a few years after the famed singer. At Rochester Adams High School, the pressure on students to wear preppy clothes with certain labels was relentless. In this elite suburban enclave, my sister learned that dressing for success and carefully cultivating one's personal image can open doors that otherwise remain closed to even the brightest students. Today, Nancy is an attorney at one of the nation's leading law firms—and Madonna is one of the wealthiest women in the world. In both cases, though the style of clothes each wore was very different, they did make the difference.

Without divulging any more gory details, my sisters' and my experiences with clothes, compulsive shopping, weight control, dating, charge cards, sexual harassment, and the body-image blues could fill an entire volume on the subject of the beauty culture's dangers. Beauty—the kind that's designed, packaged, advertised, and sold at a profit by countless manufacturers, models, media moguls, and merchandisers across the country each day—doesn't come cheap. And the havoc it wreaks in our lives is an ugly picture.

Under Our Skin

Though beauty-related issues aren't the only source of such problems, they can certainly be a contributing factor. That's because cultural beliefs about beauty don't just define how we should look; they also powerfully influence many of our most important experiences—including mate selection, school performance, friendship choices, and job status.[9]

Christians aren't exempt from these pressures. Whether we're waiting in line at the grocery store, driving to work, or walking through a shopping mall, we're bombarded with photographic images of impossibly beautiful, incredibly thin women. Consequently, it's challenging not to worry about the way others view us.

We know we shouldn't be concerned with "worldly" things, and yet we live in the world. So we look in the mirror and wonder what more we can do to improve our complexion, whiten our teeth, and change our hair. We step on the scales and inwardly moan to discover that holiday eating has added four pounds. When we try on a bathing suit, we notice every extra ounce of flesh protruding in the wrong places and wonder if liposuction might help.

Even at church, we're confronted by countless reminders of the beauty industry: L'Oréal lipstick and Maybelline mascara, professionally manicured nails and home-highlighted hair, Leslie Fay dresses and Levi jeans.

One friend of mine tells me she spends nearly 90 minutes styling her hair on Sunday mornings; another admits to regularly locking herself in the bathroom to ensure every bit of makeup is in place before leaving for weekly worship. I don't think either of these women are unusual; in fact, they're a lot like you and me.

In years past, when my two teenage daughters and I tried to get ready for church at the same time, we sometimes managed to blow fuses—the result of three hairdryers overloading the circuits. Then—*voilá*—the big moment would finally arrive, and my daughters and I would casually march out the door, leaving a cough-inducing cloud of cologne and hair spray in our wake. My husband, waiting in the car, failed to see any humor in this weekly event. He would periodically honk the horn to remind us he was ready to go—and had been for a long time.

Sometimes waiting for a church service to begin is a

lot like watching a department store fashion show. Each immaculately dressed, color-coordinated woman walks down the aisle and slides into her seat. Any Sunday is bad enough, but the fashion show becomes even more obvious on Easter Sunday.

It's not unusual for those in the sanctuary to make observations each week. I know, because, like you, I've made them: "Wow, look at the dress Cindy has on!" "That hand-knit sweater Martha's wearing is really attractive. Who made it?" "Look at Carol's new fur coat—isn't it wild?" "Can you believe Janet bought those shoes on sale for only 24 dollars?" "Since when did Judy start wearing hats?"

It's a fact: unless we've dropped out of popular culture altogether (which a few exceptional women—such as Mother Teresa and many generations of faithful Amish women—have), our appearances tend to mirror the culture in which we live as surely as our bathroom mirrors reflect our natural, God-given appearance. Erma Bombeck speaks for many of us when she comments:

> Here's my morning ritual. I open a sleepy eye, take one horrified look at my reflection in the mirror and then repeat with conviction: "I'm me and I'm wonderful. Because God doesn't make junk." [10]

Now for the million dollar question: whose mirror are we more comfortable with—our culture's or our Creator's? And which reflection are we relying on most? Like Mrs. Bombeck, are we trying to convince ourselves of something we say with our minds, but can't quite believe deep down in our hearts?

I suspect many of you have had the same questions I've had about beauty. What is real beauty? Where does it come from? Does virtue produce physical attractiveness? Does it matter to God if I color my hair, worry about my weight, or have liposuction done? Are there any scriptural standards I should follow concerning beauty? To what degree am I responsible for not making others stumble— including men—by my appearance? And why is it that what I see with my spiritual eyes concerning beauty and how I act are so often in opposition?

I think I'm pretty typical of many Christian women when I struggle between the way God made me and the way I sometimes wish I'd been made; between the way I picture myself looking and how I actually look; between what others expect me to do about my appearance and what the Lord expects of me. In other words, I'm not completely comfortable with my culture *or* my appearance—I sometimes battle both.

Wrestling and Winning

Is the battle I'm engaged in simply a symptom of double-mindedness? I don't think so. Perhaps it's more indicative of the kind of struggle the Apostle Paul was talking about when he wrote: "I do not understand what I do. For what I want to do I do not do, but what I hate I do. . . . For I have the desire to do what is good, but I cannot carry it out." [11]

As long as I participate in America's affluence and live inside my body, I'll continue to wrestle to some degree with social expectations of what I eat and wear, what cosmetics I use, how I do my hair, how much I weigh, and how I look at others—things that nearly all Americans, if we're honest with ourselves, struggle with every day to a greater or lesser extent. The decisions, comparisons, and temptations you and I face concerning beauty aren't going to go away once and for all. Period! It comes with the territory of being a particular type of earthbound creature called a "contemporary American woman."

Yet, despite this, we needn't be psychologically, physically, or spiritually trapped by beauty. For Christians, the worship of beauty is simply not an option.

The ancient Greek notion that "what is beautiful is also good" isn't biblical. In fact, the relationship of physical attractiveness to spiritual beauty is far more precarious than many of us realize. "There is a strong belief that what is beautiful is also good," says Dr. Rita Freedman in *Beauty Bound*. "We may give lip service to so-called higher moral values and dutifully insist that beauty lies within, that looks are superficial, and that character is what counts. But such sanctimonious maxims only cover up a strong unconscious worship of appearance."[12]

As with any other spiritual trap, we do well to remember that the Lord kindly provides a way out of this situation.[13] In terms of today's beauty culture, this lies, first of all, in understanding what we're up against. Second, our escape lies in *continually turning to God—not to our culture or ourselves—as the true source of our identity.*[14] As Paul does in the epistle to the Romans, we can confidently proclaim the source of our liberty—the Lord Jesus Christ—even in the midst of this struggle![15]

By examining beauty more closely and making conclusions based on a study of Scripture, we can learn how to re-interpret the power and meaning of beauty in new ways.

After you've finished reading this book, you will have gained the information, biblical resources, spiritual encouragement, and practical ideas that will enable you to find greater freedom and meaning in being the woman God is creating you to be.

The Power of Beauty

At my son David's high school last year, one of his classmates, a stunning-looking blonde senior named Shannon Pine, reached success as a model by appearing in *Seventeen* magazine, on the cover of *Sassy*, and in Macy's newspaper ads. She also had the full attention of her classmates because she drove a top-of-the-line sports car. But I noticed that it wasn't only the guys gawking at this willowy beauty; she was the focus of her female classmates' attention as well. Her clothes, hairstyle, and make-up were a popular target of conversation—and unabashed stares—among the young women who envied Shannon's sleek style.

What is it about physical female beauty that holds women and men alike by its power? I'm convinced women's physical attractiveness *does* have power— enough to alter people's lives and affect the course of history. Consider the biblical stories of Sarah and Abraham, Rachel and Jacob, Bathsheba and David, and Esther and Xerxes, for example.[16] In each case, a woman's external appearance directly influenced not only the men who were drawn to it, but the future of the world as well. (We'll look in-depth at these stories in chapter 7.)

Today, the international beauty industry exploits the power of beauty for an enormous profit. Some of our own histories have been changed by it as well.

Whether we acknowledge it or not, women's physical beauty has the power to create an intense yearning and spiritual restlessness in both men *and* women. Christians' discussions on sex, beauty, and lust characteristically center on women as the objects of men's desire. What is usually overlooked, however, is that feminine beauty can also be the object of *women's* desire as well: *the desire to be physically beautiful and to possess what is physically beautiful for one's self.*

This urge can be as powerfully captivating as any other kind of lust, and every bit as spiritually devastating. Acceptance of current beauty ideals filters into the innermost parts of our identity—the way we think about ourselves and see those around us, how we act and feel, the manner in which we live out our sexuality and our approach to the sexuality of others. It can range from an underlying heart attitude to a full-blown, self-destructive soul obsession.

This may sound somewhat overstated or a little odd. It seemed that way to me at first, too. But God never fails to change our way of seeing ourselves as we seek to know Him better. The Lord is jealous for us and desires that we turn our hearts toward worshiping, serving, and loving Him above everything and everyone else. Even when we fail God in this regard, we can always count on this: our Father in heaven is continually working within us to conform us to the image of His Son, Jesus Christ. It's a promise: "The one who calls you is faithful and he will do it." [17]

Reflex Reactions?

How many of us can say we're *totally* free from beauty-related envy and lust—coveting the beauty of others for ourselves? I'm certainly not. The good news is that as I uncover its destructive web of influence in my life, I find myself increasingly crying out to Christ to untangle me. It doesn't take an expert to tell me that looks-obsession is rampant in our society, and, like most women of my generation, I'm not immune to it.

Let me illustrate. Recently, I noticed Phil Donahue had scheduled a panel of women on his show to talk about breast implants. Knowing it would be a helpful part of my research, I tuned in on that particular morning.

While watching the program, I was somewhat surprised when one of the guests, a plastic surgeon, showed before and after photographs of women's breasts to demonstrate how surgical reconstruction can enhance one's appearance. The final picture displayed an extremely small-chested woman who, after surgery, had two perfectly shaped size C breasts. The change was more than dramatic—it was absolutely astounding.

I guarantee plenty of women watching the show stared at the picture of those beautifully shaped breasts, not looking at the photographs with sexual desire, but because they were considering what it would be like to have breasts like that of their own. Few women in my age group would have failed to at least flirt with the idea of breast reconstruction after witnessing such an appealing promotion of cosmetic surgery.

What I find particularly troubling is that in spite of my

own good judgment, I found myself, if only for a moment, considering how nice it would be to have such fabulous breasts (that is, until I watched the rest of the show and heard about the possible effects of silicone implants). But my ability to rationalize away the desire didn't undo my initial reaction. I responded as if with a reflex reaction to contemporary beauty ideals and expectations.

One Woman's Story

A few weeks later a friend and I were discussing this particular Donahue show over tea. She confided to me that her grandmother, her mother, and she all had chosen to have their breasts surgically enlarged. Not only was it considered the normal thing to do, her family simply expected her to have the procedure done. And so, about the time she was graduating from high school, she went to the same surgeon who had performed her mother's and grandmother's surgery. Only her best friend knew.

"Before, when I would try on bathing suits or dresses, the tops always looked baggy, like they needed filling out," shared my friend. "My mother's offer was so kind, really. She wanted to give that to me. But now I'm considering having the implants taken out. I worry about whether they're safe or not. I'm also concerned about having more surgery to undo this. I'm not sure what I'm going to do."

I empathize with my friend. Totally! Although I've never had cosmetic surgery, its availability lurks in my mind, only occasionally leaping into view—like when I am buying new lingerie for a weekend getaway with my husband. Just knowing liposuction, chin tucks, and abdomen flattening exist tempts me to consider changing my appearance even though I'm rationally against it.

It's all right to want to look nice—to care about our bodies and physical appearance. The danger comes when these things become a central concern, dominating the way we see ourselves and others. We're all vulnerable to being pulled back and forth between what we know in our minds about God's good design for our lives and how we feel about ourselves due to the beliefs and values imbued in our culture. Some women may have resolved this inner struggle completely. I haven't yet, nor have most of my friends. So why is it so difficult for us to accept ourselves the way God made us?

Discerning Hidden Desires

While some of the struggle is simply due to a fallen human nature bent on self-centeredness, it's also due to our society's beliefs about beauty. Like my friend who, as a teenager, was influenced by her family's beauty expectations, we *all* face the pressure of an everywhere-we-look cultural mandate equating physical attractiveness with "what is good." *The high value our culture places on being beautiful makes it all the more appealing to think about ways to become more attractive ourselves.*

Take, for example, the *Sports Illustrated Swimsuit Issue.* You may be unfamiliar with this annual American media event—and I'm certainly not recommending that you run out and find a copy—but suffice it to say that the *SISI* epitomizes our culture's obsession with female physical perfection. By presenting about a half-dozen of the world's most alluring bathing beauties posed exotically in one of the world's most fabulous tropical locations, millions of these magazines are sold. (Understandably, most normal-looking women resent this.)

While I can understand why men unabashedly pore over this annually awaited pictorial display, *women* also casually pick up the magazine, leaf through it, and sometimes actually buy it. According to the magazine, sales among women triple for the swimsuit issue: readership jumps to 41 million, including 14 million women, for the special edition of *Sports Illustrated* published each February.[18] Why?

I believe that while men may fantasize about possessing a woman's beauty by "conquering" it sexually, we women fantasize about possessing beauty by *imitating* and *acquiring* it in order to become more beautiful and sexually alluring ourselves.

Most women, Christian or not, have acquired the habit of measuring their own looks against the looks of other women. For many of us, it's something we think about quite a lot—a socially-sanctioned, media-manipulated desire we rarely put a name on, but one that consumes and distorts our God-given, true selves just as powerfully as sexual lust does.

If a beautiful, well-groomed, attractively dressed woman with a fantastic figure and gorgeous hair walks into a room full of people, what happens? It isn't just men who look at and desire her beauty. The gaze of almost every other woman in the room is riveted on her. *They look at and desire her beauty, too!*

Most women don't lust after men's bodies in the same

way that men lust after women's bodies. (We even tend to think of it as being beneath us to stoop to this kind of raw erotic lust.) But isn't *our* unique brand of lust—the secret inner desire with which we enviously gaze at women's magazines, diet food commercials, our favorite movie actresses, and attractively attired women at church—simply lust directed from a different angle?

Targeted for Exploitation

In case I haven't convinced you yet, here's one last illustration. In the Sunday paper yesterday, there was a soap advertisement showing a clean-scrubbed woman in a white satin negligee. She was provocatively exposing as much smooth skin and ample cleavage as possible, smiling eye-to-eye toward the intended reader. But who *is* the typical reader of a coupon-carrying ad for bath soap? My educated guess is that it isn't a *he* but a *she*—a woman between the ages of 25 and 45 to whom the manufacturer wants to appeal with a simple message: "If you use our soap, you can look as sexy as this woman." Interesting, isn't it, when you really think about it?

Today's beauty industry exploits and manipulates women's tendency toward covetousness and envy of beauty just as the international pornography industry exploits and manipulates men's visual tendency toward sexual lust.[19] For too long, we've focused on keeping *Playboy* and *Penthouse* out of our homes for the sake of our men without seriously considering the effect distorted beauty ideals have on us. How else can we explain our obsessions and failure to deal with them?

While we're understandably outraged by the pornography epidemic, the allure of beauty offers a much more subtle brand of temptation for women. When we become Christians, we aren't automatically exempt from being taken hostage by the beauty ideals of our society. We're not "delivered" from worrying about how we look and how others see us. (Now, wouldn't that be something? To never worry about our appearance again? That really *would* be a miracle!)

Rather than offering life-giving alternatives to our culture, however, we're more likely to substitute a Christianized version of beauty-related behaviors for the more worldly variety. Consequently, many of us are still caught up in trying to be thin and pretty in order to feel good about ourselves. We're still trying to impress others in the same way we were before becoming believers. But is this the Lord's best for us?

Life doesn't have to be this way: it's too heavy a yoke to bear, and besides, it's not what God intends for us at all. Instead, as we live as both creatures of our culture *and* as children of God, we can choose to lighten the load of today's burdensome beauty expectations by wholeheartedly embracing the *best* kind of beauty—the kind that comes when we find our true identity in the character and image of Jesus Christ.

A. W. Tozer once wrote that people can be known by what they think about most, what they desire most, how they use their money and their leisure time, what they laugh at, who and what they admire, and the company they keep. For many of us, issues related to weight, hair, clothing, sexual attractiveness, and our overall appearance take up too much energy and mental focus in each of these areas, though we may be loathe to admit it.

If you find yourself struggling—as I do—with taming the beauty monster and keeping this beast in its proper place, the next few chapters will be of special interest to you.

Action Plan

A Quick Self-Check Test

Here is a self-check test to help you evaluate how you feel about your appearance.

Reflect for a moment on how your total appearance— your weight, clothes, hairstyle, mannerisms, facial expressions, and body language—has been shaped by what you value and by those around you. How important is your appearance to you? How often do you think about it? How much money do you spend on it? How do you feel about your weight? How conscious are you of your appearance when you're around other people?

To help you evaluate these questions, use this simple, not-too-serious, and completely nonacademic self-check test. All you need to do is choose the answer for each question that comes closest to your own current experience. Then fill in the points to discover how preoccupied you are with beauty issues. (If more than one answer applies, select the one with the *highest* point total.)

1. I've dieted to lose weight during the last
____ 24 hours (10 points)
____ month (5 points)
____ year (1 point)
____ decade (0 points)

2. I look at other women's appearances and compare myself to them
____ almost always (10 points)
____ frequently (5 points)
____ rarely (1 point)
____ never (0 points)

3. I normally weigh myself
____ more than once a day (10 points)
____ daily (5 points)
____ several times a week (3 points)
____ weekly (2 points)
____ monthly (1 point)
____ annually or only at medical check-ups (0 points)

4. When I'm in public without any makeup on, I feel
____ ugly (10 points)
____ naked, invisible, or below potential (5 points)
____ plain (1 point)
____ no differently than if I am wearing makeup (0 points)

5. I worry about my weight and/or my appearance
____ once an hour or more (10 points)
____ off and on throughout the day (5 points)
____ a few times a week (1 point)
____ hardly ever (0 points)

6. Almost every time I eat, at least once, I usually think about
____ how much I should weigh or how fat I am (10 points)
____ the number of fat grams/calories I'm consuming
      (5 points)
____ ways to satisfy my hunger appropriately (1 point)
____ enjoying and being thankful for my meal (0 points.)

7. When I look in the mirror, I typically see
____ every imperfection (10 points)

____ several imperfections (5 points)
____ a few imperfections (1 point)
____ me (0 points)

Total points ____

If you scored over 50 points, you're a full-fledged participant in the beauty game. Cultural ideals and expectations about beauty have a major impact on your identity, deeply influencing the way you see yourself—as well as the way you see others.

If you scored 21-49 points, you're a half-hearted participant/observer in the beauty game. While beauty issues are still important to you, it's likely that you're already making compromises to lessen the impact of current beliefs about beauty on your walk with God.

If you scored 5-20 points, you're a reluctant observer/participant in the beauty game. Beauty's ability to harm people hasn't escaped your attention: as a result, you've taken a number of serious steps to decrease your level of involvement in today's beauty market.

If you scored less than 5 points, you don't participate in or even observe the beauty game. You're either a missionary living in a remote region of Bangladesh or have dropped out of mainstream society altogether.

After taking this test for the first time, I was somewhat surprised at how high my own point total was—an indication of my preoccupation with the beauty culture and my near-automatic response to it. This realization brought conviction and the courage to change.

❧ *Focus Questions* ❧

1. Do you often feel judged according to how you look? If so, how do you respond?

2. Given our culture's heavy emphasis on physical attractiveness, in what ways have you been most influenced by today's beauty ideals and expectations?

3. How would your life change if you never had to think or worry about your appearance—clothes, cosmetics, facial expressions, size, hairstyle, etc.—again?

❧ Two ❧

The Cult of Image

Every time I get dressed and look in the mirror, the battle begins: This dress makes my hips look huge. These pants are too tight. This sweater makes me look lumpy. Tight shirts just show how flat-chested I am. I can't wear short short sleeves, my arms are chunky. Turtlenecks make my double chin stand out. . . . I'm not alone in this. My friend Joyce, whose size-four shape I would kill for, constantly complains that her thighs resemble large frozen hams. Marge, my reed-thin aerobic instructor, swears she has a potbelly, although no one has been able to find it. I'll bet even Michelle Pfeiffer spent hours in her dressing room saying, "I can't possibly wear the Catwoman outfit. It makes my rear end look like a trailer." When it comes to body image, women just can't see straight.

— *Tamara Eberlein*, First for Women,
15 March 1992

Beware of despairing about yourself; you are commanded to put your trust in God, and not in yourself.

— *St. Augustine, 354 A.D.*

There's no doubt about it. Throughout the world, each culture creates and defines its own ideal of feminine beauty. Pondering this, fashion editor Judith Newman recently wrote in *Mirabella* magazine:

> The day I decided to have the fat sucked out of my body, I saw a documentary about a coming-of-age ritual for girls in the Niger Delta: fifteen- to seventeen-year-olds are secluded for three weeks and forced to do nothing but eat. The idea is that they need extra flesh on their bodies to attract a man and prepare for motherhood. As I dialed the plastic surgeon, I couldn't help thinking: Who can escape being a product— a sometime-victim—of her culture?[1]

While reading these comments, I was reminded of a close friend of my mother's whom I'll call Margaret. Margaret's husband had passed away when she was in her early 40's. Unexpectedly forced into a full-time job and its associated dating pressures, Margaret began paying a considerable amount of attention to her appearance. With three older children—two had already graduated from high school—Margaret longed for greater financial stability and a husband's daily companionship. A number of years later, she married her second husband, Bill, and they moved to a beautiful house on the other side of the city.

Margaret had always paid attention to her body,

though the focus intensified when she wanted to remarry. She stayed fit, strictly controlled her eating, and took a great deal of pride in her youthful appearance. Yet her abdomen sagged, and Bill often teased Margaret about it. No matter how much she exercised and dieted, her stomache stubbornly refused to firm up. When she turned 55, Margaret decided to have cosmetic surgery to fix the "problem," rationalizing that it would be well worth the cost: $2,500 for the surgery, and six weeks of recovery as her abdominal muscles healed.

I visited Margaret a week after her operation. She couldn't stand up straight because it hurt so much, and grimaced every time she laughed or sneezed. Looking back, I clearly remember thinking how sad it was that Margaret had put herself through so much pain just to look a little bit better. I'd never even noticed that her abdomen was flabby! Later, I heard her husband still complained about her appearance. It made me ache to think that she chose to suffer physically rather than find a more lasting way to make peace with her body and her husband.

The High Price of Beauty

Because our attitudes about beauty are cultural and, therefore, controllable, it's encouraging to realize that we don't have to buy into the lie that says we're worth less when our looks don't measure up. Even so, why is it so much more difficult for us to deal with our vulnerability to the allure of beauty ideals today than it was for women 50 years ago?

Perhaps, it's because the pressures women face have never been greater, even though envy is as old as Eve.

Since the 1960s, there's been a titanic explosion in the manufacturing and marketing of beauty. According to British historian Dr. Arthur Marwick, it wasn't until the sixties that physical beauty became "an autonomous status characteristic" with an intrinsic value of its own.[2]

During this period, a truly unique phenomenon took place in our society. As accelerated modernization in Western culture stimulated an unprecedented appetite for beauty, advances in technology simultaneously expanded the availability of beauty-related goods and services. Consequently, the way women naturally looked suddenly seemed downright unappealing compared to how they could look, for the right price.

Capitalizing on the cult of self-worship set off in the sixties, the beauty industry continues to feed our preoccupation with scales and mirrors. Dr. Marwick perceptively points out:

> All around us lies the evidence that our civilization, as it exists now, has an intense preoccupation with personal appearance and gives a very high rating to human beauty. Whether on the billboards which line our streets and stations, in the glossy magazines which jostle for position on the bookstalls and in the newsagents, or during the regular assaults of television commercials on our own living rooms, we see that the received method of marketing products of every type is to associate them with a beautiful human being.[3]

Each year, billions of dollars are paid into the beauty industry by everyday people like us: $20 billion on cosmetics, $2 billion on hair products, $800 million on feminine hygiene products, $300 million on cosmetic surgery, $33 billion to the diet industry, and a whopping $74 billion on diet foods.[4] A hefty portion of these revenues, in turn, are shrewdly invested in advertising all these products.

Is it any wonder we feel fat and ill at ease with ourselves if we're the slightest bit too heavy or, if we look particularly nice, that we're self-conscious about our appearance and its effect on others?

A Historic Comparison

Sometimes I imagine what it must have been like for one of my ancestors, possibly living as an illiterate peasant in preindustrial Europe. What if she were to catch a rare glimpse of a pretty noblewoman riding by in a carriage, or look up at a great-looking princess during some sort of royal swearing-in ceremony? For an ancestor of mine, an event like this was likely to be a once-in-a-lifetime exposure to affluent beauty culture.

This ancestor didn't have to walk by shelves attractively displaying hundreds of the latest beauty products at her local grocery store on her way to the dairy case; she milked her own cow. There were no billboards along the highways, and, besides, she never left town. Her tiny thatched-roof cottage didn't house a TV, radio, VCR, or CD player—she didn't have electricity. She never purchased a women's magazine or Sunday newspaper filled with beautiful models. More than likely, she didn't have a hairbrush, never used soap, had no mirror, owned one pair of homemade shoes, and wore a simple, hand-sewn, tunic-like garment which hung loosely around her ample figure. She didn't have a bathroom scale, either.

I'm sure that this woman could have recognized physical beauty, if she'd ever glimpsed it, but there weren't many opportunities. Her plain features never knew the feel of frosted lipstick nor the texture of translucent powder. The look of her face and her body did not define or determine her social status: that was determined by her parents', and later her husband's, position in the community.

As Dr. Marwick eloquently explains, beauty as an everyday concern for all but the wealthiest members of society was unheard of until relatively recently:

> From classical times till at least the late nineteenth century the overwhelming majority of the inhabitants of the West scratched a living from the land. They were mobile neither geographically nor socially: the peasant lived, worked, married and died within [her] own community. For neither man nor woman was there much choice in the way of sexual partners: the notion of choosing someone because of their superior personal appearance was an almost meaningless one. Standards of nutrition and health were low and so also, therefore, were sex drives: marriage was overwhelmingly a matter of stern practicality rather than of sexual gratification. Again, therefore, personal appearance was scarcely a matter of great concern. Even had private inclination existed, without the chance to travel, without the chance to move up in society, the opportunity for comparison, and therefore for selection, scarcely existed. . . . Even for the highest born, life was brutish and potentially short: every sinew had to be stretched towards maintaining and, if possible, improving family fortunes.[5]

In our society, this has all changed, of course. (Obviously, some of it for the better and, perhaps not so obviously, some of it for the worse.) *Today, the way a woman looks is considered to be one of her most defining personal features, as well as her leading sexual and economic asset.* Subsequently, as long as she's an active participant in American culture, she'll be reminded of her inadequacies at almost every turn.

Media, Magazines, and Megabucks

Unlike my ancestor of yore, I've seen images of thousands of beautiful women in my lifetime. A number of significant beauty-related statistics have shaped my own unique cultural experience as an American woman in the late twentieth century. Consider:

• The average American television viewer sees about 650 TV commercials each week—their personal share of the 1,000 ads broadcast each day.[6]

• In 1989 alone, the advertising revenue for toiletries and cosmetics paid to magazines came to $650 million, a figure 10 times higher than the income obtained from ads for cleaning products.[7]

• Each month, 18 million men in the United States buy one or more of the 165 different pornographic magazines; one in every ten American men reads *Playboy*, *Penthouse* or *Hustler* on a monthly basis.[8]

• Popular women's magazines on the newsstands offering a sensual slant on women have also grown in recent years, with names like *Self, New Woman, Elle,* and *Allure.* From *Glamour* to *Redbook* to *Cosmopolitan,* women's beauty (and sexuality) is packaged and sold, with women the targeted buyers. These magazines, and their masculine counterparts, all create, define, and market idealized images of women as the current social standard of beauty.

• Today's average model, dancer, or actress is thinner than 95 percent of the female population.[9] A generation ago, the average model weighed eight percent less than the average American woman; she now weighs 23 percent less.[10]

• In a study of changes in five popular American magazines from 1960-1979—*Ladies' Home Journal, Vogue, Time, Playboy,* and *Ms.*—researchers found that fully 77 percent of the women pictured in ads appeared to be under 30, while only

37 percent of the men were that age. Less than 2 percent of the models were in their 60s; by 1979, the average age of models decreased significantly for every magazine except *Time*—even as the age of subscribers was increasing.[11]

According to today's image cult, I'm to be as pretty as possible if I hope to succeed professionally or sexually in today's world. My nails are to have no chips, cracks, or ridges; my lips must never be chapped or too pale; my complexion is to be as zit-less, grease-less, and pit-less as possible, with wrinkles, crow's feet, unsightly hair, dry spots, moles, freckles, and smile lines kept to an absolute minimum; my teeth must not be yellow or crooked or uneven; my hair should be cut to complement my facial structure and conditioned to shine, bounce, curl, and not get frizzy; my body should match widely published dimensions for its height and frame-size while strictly controlled at all times—especially in regards to eating and exercising; and I'm to passionately dislike any flab or cellulite on my body so much, that I'm willing to cut or starve myself to get rid of it.

Once I've bought into this idea of beauty, there are countless products and services available to help me attain it, thanks to today's multibillion dollar beauty industry. The problem is, *I never seem to be able to obtain the image they're selling me!*

The Family Circle Survey

In 1990 *Family Circle* reported the results of an extensive survey on how American women feel about their looks.[12] Since it comes from "the horse's mouth," so to speak, the *Family Circle* survey is an accurate barometer of just how many of us are struggling with today's media-promoted, age-targeted, strategically-marketed beauty blitz.

Not surprisingly, the survey found that most women are fed up with the expectations of today's beauty culture, yet still feel like they don't measure up. Of the many *Family Circle* readers who responded, the majority said they:

1. Think they're too fat.

2. Believe that younger is better.

3. Like their faces better than any other body part.

4. Are reluctant to wear a bathing suit.

5. Blame their parents—not advertisers—for their skewed self-perceptions.

6. Treat other women more kindly about their appearance than they do themselves.

7. Criticize the way women look much more harshly than men do.[13]

One respondent's comment echoes the *why-do-we-do-this-when-we're-smart-enough-to-know-better?* frustration millions of American women feel so keenly today: "I'm tired of the 'perfect woman' represented through TV, movies and magazines," admitted Jana Gleim, a 37-year-old mother of three from a small town in western Nebraska. "Because we can't measure up—an impossible expectation—we're made to feel we've somehow failed ourselves, our families, and society."

She then added, "In your head you know it's unrealistic to imitate a size-seven model, but in your heart you'd like to look the way she does."[14]

Sixty percent of women in the United States wear a size 12 or larger, and a significant number—31 percent, or a total of 35 million—are size 16 or over.[15] The average American woman today weighs 146 pounds. The average model or actress weighs 23 percent less, is under age 25, wears the best clothing money can buy, and is paid large bucks to sell us something (cigarettes, a big-budget movie, or *Wheel of Fortune*). Of course we want to look like her, but we have a hard time achieving this goal. Like the *Family Circle* survey respondents, we end up with a continual sense of failure.

Remember Barbie?

On posters promoting the film *Pretty Woman*, amazingly slender, minimally dressed Julia Roberts (as Hollywood's Happiest Hooker) is teasingly pictured standing back-to-back against Richard Gere (the Fine-Looking Financier), leading him away by his very expensive designer silk tie. But guess what? Not even Julia Roberts had a good enough body for the ad: her head was superimposed on the body of an anonymous woman! In the opening scene of the movie, again, it isn't Roberts' body we see sprawled out on the bed, but a model's.

If not even Julia Roberts can look the way she's "supposed" to, how can we? Impossible images, indeed.

"Women strive for a high degree of physical perfection and magnify their flaws into failings that merit self-hate because our whole culture has been seduced by the idea of physical perfectibility," reports Roberta Pollack Seid in *Never Too Thin: Why Women Are At War with Their Bodies*. "What has been displaced is not only our sense of what constitutes normal eating but also what constitutes normal bodies."[16]

Each culture has its own perception of the ideal human figure. This ideal changes over time and is directly influenced by cultural beliefs. Today, because of the myriad images we see in magazines, movies, music videos, television shows, and product commercials, the ideal body is that of a model. But besides these influences, millions of us also grow up playing with fashion dolls.

As the most popular doll of all time, Barbie has had a lasting impact on our culture. I should know: I was the first on my block to own one. Barbie, Ken, Midge, and Skipper were my make-believe companions for the majority of my grade-school years. Collecting clothes and accessories for them was my premier extracurricular occupation from 1959-1964. (If I only knew where all that stuff is now, it would probably be worth a fortune.) Recently, it was said of Barbie: "She's a fantasy object for men for little girls, if that makes sense." [17] In other words, she's a doll designed according to an adult man's imagination—not dreamed up by someone's five-year-old daughter—then sold as a playmate to young girls. I remember wanting to be Barbie, with her teeny waist, big breasts, and incredibly long, thin legs. Today, I wonder what impact my imaginary friends might have had on my developing identity and beauty ideals. I wonder, as well, if my imaginary friends have impacted the way I feel about my body today.

I recently ran into an interesting analysis of what the averaged figure of 15 fashion dolls translates into in reality. By assigning the dolls a five-foot-six-inch height, it was determined that the bust measurement would range from 26.4 to 32.0 inches, the waist from 17.0 to 23.3 inches, and the hips from 26.9 to 32.3 inches. But when the dolls' bust measurements were standardized to 36 inches, their heights climbed to between 6-foot-2-inches and 7-foot-5 inches! As a result, researchers concluded that no healthy individual could possibly have the extreme proportions of Barbie dolls.[18]

Barbie's maker, Mattel, claims Barbie was designed as an aspirational role model. But what are children to aspire *to*? An unnaturally short-waisted, long-legged, curvaceous beauty made of plastic—or a seven-foot tall, size-three Norwegian giant? Just what every girl needs to strive for, right? Wrong.

Now, 30 years after Barbie's arrival, tall, unreasonably thin models and performers stalk runways, stages, and movie screens in true Barbie style. "A woman's appearance is now dependent on how closely she approximates Barbie," says Pauline Bart, a sociologist at the Univeristy of Illinois in Chicago. "You're supposed to be very thin with large breasts. This is difficult." [19]

Tearing Up Paper Tigers

In a United Nations report on the status of women, what do you think was cited by a panel of experts as the worst offender in stereotyping women as sex objects and making them feel they are an inferior class through the degradation of their bodies? Was it pornography? Prostitution? MTV? Not surprisingly, *advertising* topped the list—an important fact for us to remember when we are depressed about our appearance.

Commenting on this tough truth, journalist Naomi Wolf wonders: "Why do women react so strongly to nothing, really—images, scraps of paper? Is their identity so weak? Why do they feel they must treat 'models'—mannequins—as if they were 'models'—paradigms? Why do women react to the 'ideal,' whatever form she takes at the moment, as if she were a non-negotiable commandment?" [20]

The good news is we don't have to. If we're feeling dissatisfied with ourselves and worn out by the world's brand of beauty, let's make that the beginning of something *really* beautiful—our willingness to let the Lord mold and shape us, for His glory, according to the model our Maker chooses for our lives. According to 1 Samuel 16:7, "Man looks at the outward appearance, but the Lord looks at the heart." It's time we started believing it!

Action Plan

Step off the Judgment Seat

If you often think something's wrong with the way you look, you can find healing through redirecting your mindset.

• Remember, opinions about beauty are primarily shaped by one's culture and family. Because of the cult of image that exists in our society today, we need to continually protect ourselves from statements that tell us we're "bad" if we don't look perfect, or that we've done something "wrong" if our appearance doesn't match the mannequins in shopping mall windows.

• Ask yourself if the messages you're receiving about the way you look are mainly positive or negative. Are they causing you to judge yourself unfairly?

• Encourage yourself by considering the virtues and values Christ exemplified. He taught us to be kind, gentle, hopeful, gracious, patient, joyful, loving, simple, honest, and true. Resist the temptation to heap scorn, desperation, and hatred upon yourself (or others) concerning your body's appearance.

• Ask God to change your heart and how you feel about your body. Huge hips, flat chests, wide waists, chunky arms, double chins, large thighs, potbellies, and big buttocks are a concern for many women. If you are one of them, remember the words of St. Augustine at the beginning of this chapter and don't despair. You can learn to like and enjoy your body no matter what "shape" it's in.

Practice Telling Yourself the Truth

Temptations put forth by advertisers can be battled by reminding yourself of a few facts and recalling these three statements:

• That model looks really great, but she's also paid a vast sum of money to look that way. She and the company she works for are just trying to make me want the product she's selling. However, I don't really *want* or *need* this product.

• God loves me the way I am. I stand complete in Christ. Consequently, I can make wise choices about how to groom myself and spend my money without being sucked into this way of thinking by my culture.

• I will learn to care for and appreciate the body God has made for me. Today, I will care for and enjoy my body by:

1._____

2._____

3._____

❧ *Focus Questions* ❦

1. What is vanity?

2. Are you dissatisfied with the way you look? If so, identify several reasons why advertisers seek to create and reinforce this self-perception.

3. How might fashion dolls influence fashion and body expectations? Are they healthy or harmful toys for children to play with?

Three

Hope in a Jar

*Ladies who wish to become plump without being stout,
and have a complexion like milk and roses, cannot do
better than drink the new tea that is now all the rage in
Paris, I mean* Sterky—*which can be had at this office.
By* continually *drinking this tea, instead of the usual
tea, you will soon acquire a full bust and a complexion
on which Time will not set its ugly finger. Drink it with
milk and sugar like any other tea. You must not expect
wonders at first, but persevere and you will be pleased
with the results.*
—— *Madame Bayard,* Toilet Hints or How to Preserve
Beauty and How to Acquire It, *1883*

*Where, oh where, is the ad that promises us to be
cherished for the love we give, the kindnesses we bestow,
the generous spirit that pervades our lives? When will
the fiction that we women help create for ourselves be
supplanted by the truths we honestly live?*
—— *Lois Wyse,* Good Housekeeping, *1991*

od has given you one face, and you make yourself another," Hamlet complained to Ophelia. But could Shakespeare ever have predicted that "made up" faces would one day be as ordinary and commonplace as soap?

In the United States each year, we collectively buy 1,484 tubes of lipstick (at a cost of $4,566), 913 bottles of nail polish ($2,055), 1,324 mascaras, eyeshadows, and eyeliners ($6,849), and 2,055 jars of skin care products ($12,785) *every minute.*[1] That's $1,581,300 an hour, folks.

Today, beauty product marketing represents an almost $17 billion-per-year business in the U.S., with an annual expenditure per person of about $70, compared to $40 million in 1914—when per capita spending ran about 40 cents each year. In 1986 alone, the cosmetics stock price index rose 29 percent, compared to a 15 percent gain for the stock market as a whole.[2]

This industry depends directly on you and me, and the purchasing decisions we make every day. We help it thrive and grow. Are we investing wisely?

Before adding anything more, let me say that I wear lipstick and use mascara and brush powder on my cheeks, just as most of the women I know do. Nevertheless, I am slowly getting smarter about the choices I make. Lots smarter! And my dependence on beauty products to help me feel better about myself is diminishing daily. I've even changed my entire skin care regimen since doing research for this book—and am saving a bundle, by the way, while obtaining better results. (More on this later, I promise.)

Now when I see Lancôme's latest advertisement with Isabella ("wake up to more beautiful looking skin") Rossellini in a supposedly blissful slumber, I chuckle to myself before deciphering the lingo: *"Lancôme enters the world of Chrono-cosmetology."* Sounds pretty good, but what is it? *"At night, after facing the day's aggressions, the skin's natural biological rhythms turn to its renewal activities."* Does skin have a "rhythm," or is this just the manufacturer's sophisticated way of referring to *sleep*?

What Lancôme is *really* trying to tell me, if I decide to spend $45 for a couple of ounces of their skin treatment, is that I can expect *amazing results*. But are the actual results really that different than what I can obtain by using a cheaper product? No, they're not.

Reading between the Lines

"It's illegal for a cosmetics company to claim that its cosmetics (with the exception of those containing a sunscreen) can change, alter, or effect permanent structural change in the status of the skin—because they don't," explains consumer cosmetics expert Paula Begoun. "Cosmetics don't change the skin permanently; that's why they're called *cosmetics*. If you listen carefully, you'll see that most manufacturers don't state directly that their products cause permanent alterations—they imply it."[3]

Begoun adds that terms such as revitalize, repair, firm,

nourish, re-energize, or restore the skin are all permissible by the Food and Drug Administration, *as long as* product ingredients—such as oil or propylene glycol or mucopolysaccharides—retain water in the skin. In recent years, the FDA has outlawed blatant inaccuracies in cosmetic advertising. Yet beauty companies can still skillfully craft ads to *create the illusion* of spectacular results through indirect assertion rather than through making false promises they can't scientifically back up.

What's true for cosmetics also applies to hair products. A recent *Consumer Reports* states this in no uncertain terms.

> Shampoo cleans hair. That's all shampoo does. Hair is dead. It can't be revitalized by Nexxus Vita-Tress, fed by Jhirmack Nutribody, or treated by the folk remedy aloe vera in Halsand Agree. It can't be nourished by honey, wheat-germ oil, rosemary, chamomile, or vitamins A, E, and D, all of which are added to one brand or another, mostly to give copywriters something other than detergent to build a dream on.[4]

It's up to us consumers to discern fact from fiction. This isn't difficult: all it takes is a willingness to look beyond glossy print facades filled with high-tech terminology and fascinating faces belonging to such striking beauties as Isabella, Christy, Andie, Cindy, and Paulina, who just happen to hold huge contracts with the major cosmetics companies. It's the only way to get to the truth behind a company's multimillion dollar sales pitch—a pitch *we* ultimately finance.

Though the faces of these models may be difficult to dismiss, the terminology behind the advertising can be mastered more easily than one might think. "The words that sound scientific are often the most presumptuous and carry the least information," points out Begoun. "I've yet to find a salesperson who, when pressed, can define 'micro-refining,' 'micro-targeted,' 'micro-bubbles,' 'isotonic energy,' 'bio-synergetic,' 'bio-performance,' and 'micro-lipid-concentrate.' Often these terms have been created by the company to sound impressive, but that's about as far as it goes." [5]

A quick comparison of 20 popular skin creams heads off some of this hype. Since mass-marketed moisturizers bring in $520 million annually—a figure that doesn't include the upscale cosmetics lines—the hype part is really the *only* obvious thing about these products.[6]

The enormous difference between product prices and complex lists of ingredients tends to make us believe a Ph.D. is necessary to make smart decisions about skin care these days. Consequently, it seems much easier— and a lot more fun—to surrender to the lure of sleek packaging and simply *believe.*

By examining the primary ingredients in various products, then comparing their prices, it rapidly becomes clear that the familiar warning "buyer beware" aptly applies to any woman approaching her local cosmetics counter today.[7]

COMPARISON OF 20 SIMILAR SKIN CREAMS

Brand	Product	Price	Primary Ingredients
Almay	Vitalizing Moisture Cream	$7	Water, mineral oil, butylene glycol, propylene glycol, vegetable oil, fatty acids, squalene (shark oil), animal elastin, and synthetic beeswax.
Body Shop	Aloe Vera Moisture Cream	$7.75	Water, almond oil, glycerin, cocoa butter, thickeners, and aloe vera extract.

Borghese	Moisture Intensifier	$65	Water, cyclomethicone (a form of mineral oil), butylene glycol, olive oil, mineral oil, propylene glycol, mineral salts, flower oils (geranium, lavender, and peppermint), mucopolysaccharides, and soybean oil.
Clarins	Revitalizing Moisture Cream	$40	Water, mineral oil, thickeners, alcohols, glycerin, fatty acids, plant extracts (coneflower and horsetail), triglyceride, cholesterol, lecithin, vitamin E, sodium pca, oils (hazelnut and avocado), and vitamin B6.
Clinique	Advanced Cream	$50	Water, thickeners, glycerin, butylene glycol, squalene, fatty acids, jojoba oil, soybean oil, triglyceride, algae extract, vitamin A, and vitamin E.
Elizabeth Arden	Day Renewal Emulsion	$30	Water, squalene, propylene glycol, thickener, and lanolin.
Estee Lauder	Time Zone	$50	Water, algae extract, butylene glycol, glyceride esters (glycerin-like substances), squalene, and glycerin.
La Prairie	Cellular Night Cream	$95	Water, mineral oil, thickeners, petrolatum, and a lanolin derivative.
Lancôme	Night Renewal Cream	$45	Water, macadamia oil, glycerin, vegetable oil, cholesterol, fatty acids, serum proteins, thickeners, vitamin E, basic sugars, mucopolysaccharides, and baking soda.
L'Oréal	Plentitude Action Liposomes	$14	Water, apricot kernel oil, a form of mineral oil, animal tissue extract, glycerine, lecithin, and plant extracts.

Mary Kay	Extra Emollient Moisturizer	$9	Water, wax, squalene, sesame oil, glycerin, and soybean oil.
Neutrogena	Night Cream	$13	Water, glycerin, sesame oil, thickeners, petrolatum, vitamin B6, and cholesterol.
Oil of Olay	Moisture Replenishing Cream	$7.50	Water, mineral oil, thickeners, sunflower seed oil, sunscreen, glycerin, cholesterol, and castor oil.
Owen	Candermyl Liposome Cream	$13	Water, triglycerides, amino acids, cholesterol, glycerin, thickeners, mucopolysaccha-rides (offer the same benefit as collagen and elastin), and honey.
Pond's	Extra Thick Moisturizer	$4	Water, mineral oil, emollient, petrolatum, and thickeners.
Revlon	EuropeanCollagen Complex Cream	$14	Water, mineral oil, propylene glycol, animal collagen, sweet almond oil, thickeners, mineral oil, olive oil, lecithin, fatty acids, and lanolin oil.
Ultima II	CHR Extraordinary Cream	$65	Water, vegetable oil, mineral oil, propylene glycol, sweet almond oil, lanolin, fatty acids, glycerin, thickeners, collagen, rice bran oil, and a form of squalene.

In a Class of Their Own: Outrageously Expensive Skin Care Products Containing Unusual, But Not Necessarily Useful, Ingredients

Chanel	Skin Recovery Cream	$130	Water, amniotic fluid, propy-lene glycol, protein, and oil. (Note: There is no real proof that amniotic fluid in a cream can do anything special for skin.)

Elizabeth Arden	Ceramide Time Complex Capsules	$155	Neural lipids extract, epidermal lipids extract, and retinyl palmitrate, a derivative of vitamin A. (The extracts sound good, but there's no solid evidence that they actually do anything.)
La Prairie	Essence of Skin Caviar	$75	Water, propylene glycol, lactose (milk sugar), a form of lanolin, castor oil, panthenol (vitamin B), animal protein and placental protein. (By the way, this moisturizer costs $75 for a half-ounce. Is placental protein worth $2,400 per pound?)

After reading *Don't Go to the Cosmetics Counter Without Me*, an excellent consumer's guide to cosmetics, I decided to try the skin care regimen the author recommends.[8] To cleanse my face, I use Cetaphil Lotion ($8 for 16 ounces) which effectively removes all makeup and softens my skin. As a light "scrub" (exfoliant), I sprinkle a little baking soda ($.59 for a whole box) into the Cetaphil, or use it as a paste to lightly massage oily areas when needed. I also gently dab hydrogen peroxide ($.39 a bottle) on oily areas, blackheads, or breakouts, using a cotton pad. At night, I apply Candermyl Liposome Cream ($13) or a vitamin E cream. During the day I use a light, inexpensive moisturizer, such as Lubriderm One Step or L'Oréal Plentitude Active Daily Moisture Lotion (both around $6). When I need a mask to reduce oil, I use Philips Milk of Magnesia (under $3). There's nothing contained in costlier products that does anything more beneficial for my skin than these products do.

Cashmere Mascara and Caviar Cream

Charles Revson, the brilliant founder and financial wizard behind Revlon, understood that the key to selling beauty products to the public was actually about "selling hope, the kind that comes in a jar." Hence the hype.

But another equally powerful element adds to the marketing of the beauty mystique. Beyond the manipulation of a customer's hope for a miracle and desire for eternal youth is the inherent message that *if our product costs more, it must be better*—and that by using this highly valued product, you can *increase your own value as well.*

One of the strangest examples of this is a $14 tube of mascara by Christian Dior. Called *Thickening Lash Care with Cashmere,* it contains the sheared fur of a cashmere goat. For those who can't afford the real thing, a $1,000 cashmere sweater set, the manufacturer offers the "implied luxury," accompanied by a scientific-sounding explanation for the use of a goat's hair: "hydrolyzed cashmere—an excellent source of keratin for eyelashes." In a market that offers close to 150 kinds of mascaras, companies will try anything for a sale.[9]

Take note: a product's name, description, advertising budget, and packaging are far more valuable than the product itself.

Cosmetics marketing hasn't always been this bizarre. In the old days, sensible terms such as oil, cream, lipstick, rouge, and eyeshadow were used to describe safe stand-bys to customers. But as the year 2000 approaches, what cosmetics are called and what they contain sound more mysterious and intriguing than ever before.

In today's highly competitive and fantastically lucrative

market, we aren't only offered mascara with cashmere but also enticed with *Stress Buffer, Time Mender,* and *Liquid Crystal* skin creams; *Bio-Demaquillant,* a cleanser; *La Moda* and *Crayon Contour Des Levres* lipstick and pencil; *Creme-Gel Pour Le Contour Des Yeux* (eye cream); *Concentrato di Vita* ("Life Concentrate"—facial serum) and lipstick called *La Moda* (Borghese). And let's not forget La Prairie's sumptuous bubbles of *Skin Caviar.*

Give me a break! *All* of these products are designed to masterfully create the illusion of luxury; *none* can erase a single crow's foot or significantly alter even the smallest wrinkle on a woman's face, let alone color the eyelids or lips any better than cheaper brands can.

How else does one explain spending $90 for two ounces of moisturizer if an almost identical product can be bought for under $14—unless the customer somehow *believes* in that product's ability to perform something wondrous? Why would women buy lipstick for $17.50 in an exclusive department store when right around the corner at a discount drugstore a similar version is available for $3.85? *Because millions of us have been sold on the idea that more expensive means better.* While that may be true with other types of products and services, it certainly isn't true of cosmetics.

Interestingly, a peek at some of the corporate connections between high-end and low-end lines reveals that it's often the same companies selling both—or several—price levels of cosmetics. Understanding this effectively refutes any notion of "exclusivity" that companies carefully cultivate to boost their prices.

CORPORATE CONNECTIONS: WHO OWNS WHAT

Parent Company	*Cosmetics Lines Owned*
Cosmair	Lancôme and L'Oréal

Chesebrough Ponds	Pond's, Erno Lazlo, and Aziza
Estée Lauder	Estée Lauder, Clinique, Prescriptives, and Origins
Schering-Plough	Maybelline and Yardley of London
Proctor and Gamble	Clarion, Cover Girl, Max Factor, and Noxema
Revlon	Revlon, Almay, Borghese, Alexandra de Markoff, Charles of the Ritz, Germaine Monteil, and Ultima II
Unilever	Elizabeth Arden, Calvin Klein, and Fabergé

The good news is that in 1988, 28 percent of cosmetics were sold in supermarkets and 27 percent in drugstores. And the trend is growing.[10] Hope in a jar, perhaps—but at a discount and at fair prices. In an attempt to understand this recent trend, reporter Gretchen Morgenson asks perceptively, "Why would you drive 20 minutes to the nearest mall to pick up a bottle of Chanel nail color, when you can grab a Maybelline lacquer at your neighborhood drugstore?" [11]

In an era when high-end lipsticks are nearing $20 each, a 1.7 ounce jar of skin cream can easily cost $100, and eyeshadow may sell for close to $50, women can, in good conscience, refuse to play the game by making smart selections at the cosmetics counter. It's a good start, communicating our displeasure with such outrageous product pricing.

Do Blondes Have More Fun?

In 1991, 40 million American women spent $500 million to color their hair. Half decided to go, or stay, blonde in the process. In the same year, visits to salons for blonde services climbed 25 percent.[12] And, if this weren't enough, a recent Clairol survey tells us that among women who never color their hair, nearly 20 percent wish they were blonde.[13]

As a bottle-blonde myself, I've often reflected on such statistics and my own rationale for resorting to chemical warfare against the browning of my hair. Since I began life with a head covered with light golden curls that my mother used to tell me glistened in the sunshine, I reasoned, *Why shouldn't I be blonde now?* After all, lemon juice can only go so far toward lightening one's ever-darkening tresses, and spray-on treatments tend to turn hair orange. By around the age of 30, many women start to think they either have to do something really serious, or prepare to say good-bye to their former blondeness forever. Why not me?

I thought about it for a long time—15 years, I think. Then came the day when I finally had an appointment to officially highlight my hair—not an all-out dye job, mind you—and somehow found myself sitting through several hours of foil-wrapping, bleaching, and stinking up assorted strands of my hair.

Later that day, I was excited to pick up my husband at the airport when he returned from a business trip. I anxiously stood waiting to surprise him. I surprised him, all right! When he came through the gate and shouted "Ruby!" I realized I might have made a big mistake tampering with my hair. The next morning I rushed to another hairstylist to correct the color. It came out sort of striped, but at least the stripes were blonde, which seemed to me a step in the right direction.

That was six years ago, and I've since sat through countless "highlights" at a number of salons. I'm still not happy with my hair, and I think highlighting ranks pretty close to torture. (Hundreds of pokes and picks with a steel crochet needle in the scalp is definitely not my idea of fun at the beauty parlor.) Yet I continue to do it, because the alternatives seem very unattractive: I can't dye my hair brown without having it turn out ghastly; if I cut off all the blonde and let my natural color grow out, my hair would be an inch long, and dyeing it totally blonde wouldn't look any better—it might even look worse—and would be hard to undo if I didn't like it.

I count myself as one of the 40 million, who, if you asked us, would admit that being blonde isn't always fun, especially during the processing phase every four to eight weeks. I can freely admit it now: I was duped. Sure, one's hair looks nice when it's done right But for many of us, it's an attempt to go back to our younger days when life was more carefree. But who are we kidding, anyway? Hair coloring is one huge headache, no matter how good it makes us look.

Going for the $7,000 Glow

I realize plenty of women out there disagree with me. Consider Charla Krupp, for instance. An attractive magazine editor with highlighted blonde hair (touched up professionally every two weeks), Ms. Krupp spent exactly $7,398 beautifying her face, hair, and body in 1990.[14]

"I am not, by any stretch, the highest-maintenance woman I know," she admits, "though I've given the college tuition of my unborn child over to my hair salon, Bruno Pittini in New York. There are women who leave me in their perfumed seaweed dust with Saturday bookings for rolfing, shiatsu, mustache bleaching, head massage, foot massage, and eyebrow dyeing." [15]

Nevertheless, Charla still had to rack up her enormous beauty bill and, according to *Glamour* magazine, this is how she did it:

- manicure: $18 a week
- massage: $30 per half hour, every other week
- facial: $80, every three months
- skin care (excluding facials): $420 a year
- makeup: $612 a year
- hair color: $65, every other week
- haircut: $90, every three months
- waxing: $190 a year
- contact lenses (disposable): $360 a year
- teeth cleaning: $75, every three months
- health club: $1,298 a year
- pedicure: $25, six times a year

TOTAL: $7,398 per year

"Being a high-maintenance woman isn't for everyone," explains Krupp. "It takes an enormous amount of time, an endless supply of funds and relentless dedication to the cause of self-improvement. I don't have a hobby, so I guess this is mine. Who can put a price tag on that fabulous glow you get when you're your thinnest, your blondest, your pores their tiniest, and every inch of you is waxed all shiny and new? Certainly not I." [16]

It shouldn't stun anyone that, given the chance, millions of women congregate in beauty salons each day all around America. The "because I'm worth it" mindset is a very powerful intoxicant for women in search of comfort and affirmation. What's more, *we want to believe that when we look and feel beautiful, we'll feel better about ourselves.*

Not surprisingly, Avon's 1990 Beauty and Skin-Care Report claims that boosting self-confidence—not attracting a mate or landing a job—is the number one reason 81 percent of women give for improving their appearance. Avon offers its best beauty advice on exercise, diet, and makeup, promising, "You'll not only look good, but feel beautiful . . . every day of your life." [17] But is it really true?

Likewise, *Vogue Complete Beauty* presents what superficially appears to be a common sense plan for becoming more beautiful: "Feel beautiful and you will look beautiful. But how do you go about feeling beautiful? The answer is a circular one. You must start by looking good." [18] Sounds perfectly reasonable, doesn't it? Yet the cycle's a vicious one. Think about it. How many women do *you* know who feel beautiful based on their appearance alone?

Telling Ourselves the Truth

The fact is, the way our faces look matters, even if we would like it to be otherwise—it's the way God's designed us. British sociologist Anthony Synnott, offering a succinct summary of the human face's various roles and capabilities, explores some of the reasons why people's faces readily catch our attention.

> The face, as unique, physical, malleable, and public, is the prime symbol of the self. It is unique, for no two faces are identical, and it is in the face that we recognize each other,

and identify ourselves. Our faces are pictured in our pass-
ports and identification papers. The face is physical, and
therefore personal and intimate, yet the face is also "made
up," "put on" and subject to fashion. It is public, but also
intensely private and intimate. And malleable, with its
eighty mimetic muscles, the face is capable of over 7,000
expressions.

Furthermore, the face indicates the age, gender and
race of the self with varying degrees of accuracy, also our
health and socio-economic status, our moods and emotions, even perhaps our character and personality. The face
is also the sight of four of our five senses: sight, taste, smell
and hearing, and the site of our intakes of food drink and
air. It is also the source for non-verbal communication.
Gloria Swanson once said, "We didn't need dialogue. We
had faces." Moreover the face is also the principal determinant in the perception of our individual beauty or ugliness,
and all that these perceptions imply for self-esteem and life-
chances. The face indeed symbolizes the self, and signifies
many different facets of the self. More than any other part
of the body, we identify the face as me or you.[19]

The question we need to ask, then, is not *if* the way we
look matters to us, but how much and why. For example,
is it worth spending thousands of dollars a year to beautify
ourselves? Hundreds of dollars? How much is too much?
Where do we draw the line between paying a healthy
amount of attention to our looks and fixating on them?
Should we invest in self-beautification at all?

By finding a better basis for understanding beauty,
we'll begin to be set free from fixating on our faces and
anxiously buying into today's beauty culture. The self-
conscious glimpses in the mirror, constant comparisons
to other women, and continual faultfinding that goes
along with it will fade, because we'll discover the truth of

God's Word: that cosmetics and hair color and low body-fat percentages aren't who we really are at all.

Action Plan

Make Wise Choices

Though cosmetic companies offer countless products in every price range, we don't have to buy what they are selling. We can fight back. Here's how:

• Buy on-sale cosmetics at supermarkets and discount chains. My friend Jane says, "When I wasn't on a strict budget, I often splurged at the Clinique and Lancôme counters at Macy's, but after our baby was born, I couldn't afford to do that any longer." Jane finds that the new brands she uses compare favorably to costlier cosmetics, at greatly reduced prices. "It took a bit of experimenting to determine which products were best," she says, "but the initial investment was worth it: I save at least 60 to 75 percent on every type of cosmetic I buy. By using coupons and advertised sales, I can find comparable quality mascara and lipstick for under $4 each, when I used to spend $10 to $15."

• Don't let others pressure you to buy high-priced cosmetics. In my family buying high-priced cosmetics is the norm rather than the exception. I've often felt pressure to buy brands I couldn't afford when my sisters have raved about their latest Stendahl, Clarins, or Estée Lauder purchase. But all I have to do is think twice before seriously considering spending $30—or more—on a six-ounce bottle of soap. Because I know the ingredients of similar, less expensive products are virtually the same, I'm freed from the temptation to buy slickly packaged brands.

• If you have good reasons for preferring more expensive brands of cosmetics, stretch your buying power by choosing items only in conjunction with manufacturer's promotions that offer a "gift package" of products with minimum purchase.

• Save money by purchasing your favorite products at discount stores and supermarkets whenever possible.

• Consider trying a new skin care regimen, such as the Cetaphil and baking soda routine mentioned previously. Search for less expensive brands which will perform as well as the more expensive brands, Almay instead of Clinique, for example. Give them a try.

Though my 19-year-old daughter, Katherine, splurges on Lancôme's matte powder foundation, everything else she uses comes from a local discount store. For now, it's a nice compromise for her, and because she times her big purchases with Lancôme gift promotions, she gets what she needs as well as several free gifts.

• Just say no to all the hype. Find joy in practicing the art of understatement: clean skin, subtle lipstick, transparent powder, a bit of blush, maybe a little mascara. After applying your makeup, forget about it and go on to bigger and better things.

• Decide that as a Christian, you will offer a refreshing example others will want to emulate. Rather than imitating the images presented by our culture, point to a better hope and brighter reality—the shape of things to come.

❧ *Focus Questions* ❧

1. How much money do you spend annually on beauty? Are there any areas where you'd like to spend less, or more? What guidelines will you use to determine how much is too much?

2. What is the highest compliment you could receive concerning your appearance?

3. How can cosmetics buyers best protect themselves from being duped by product manufacturers and advertisers?

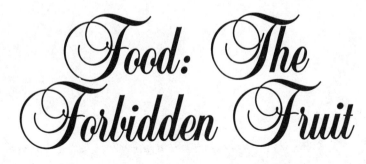

Four

Food: The Forbidden Fruit

Fat is now regarded as an indiscretion,
and almost as a crime.

—Living Age, *28 February 1914*

There's something dehumanizing about a society that says to its emerging women, "Welcome . . . but only if you look a certain way."

— *Kathy Bowen-Woodward*
Coping With a Negative Body-Image, *1989*

Almost every person I know has a love-hate relationship with food. It's rare these days to meet someone who is neither drawn to food nor repelled by it, who isn't alternately attracted to or selectively shunning temptation in the form of something like freshly baked French bread (with real butter), chocolate chip cookie dough ice cream, Black Forest cheesecake, or fettucine Alfredo. Depending on whether we're dieting or not, the endless variety of flavors, aromas, textures, and tastes associated with eating food either provokes a peak experience or a shame-inducing slump.

I can't even count the times when, at a special luncheon or dinner banquet, the topic of calories has come up at the exact moment dessert is served. Then, as I'm biting into some scrumptious concoction, an entire chorus of discordant moans and groans will chime in: *"Look at this!* How many calories do you think are in this thing? I don't even *want* to know!"

With this kind of encouragement, who'd actually eat a whole piece of peanut butter ice cream pie with Oreo cookie crust and mounds of whipped cream topping with a sprinkling of shaved chocolate, let alone more than about 10 tiny bites of the terrible thing? Not me. But, if I did eat it, do you think I'd feel okay after the deed was done?

The moral overtones associated with fatness and thinness are evidenced everywhere, with the natural enjoyment of food changed into an ongoing internal saga that never seems to quit. Whether discussed in terms of right and wrong ways to eat, or the success or failure of a specific diet, most Americans battle their appetites from one hour to the next in an effort to ward off the Great Enemy spelled F-A-T.

A National Obsession

Thinking this way about adipose tissue is neither natural nor normal: as with other beauty-related behaviors, it's a bona fide contemporary cultural phenomenon. More than any other people, we Americans are hung up on food. It's gotten so bad, in fact, that diet books outsell all other books on the market, except the Bible.

Whereas "going on a diet" was once considered a momentary interlude along life's way, dieting itself is now a way of life for millions of people in the U.S. On any given day, an estimated 25 percent of all American women are on a diet, with 50 percent finishing, breaking, or starting one.[1]

This phenomenon, of course, isn't only limited to women. Nearly *all* Americans today—some say as many as 90 percent—believe they're overweight.[2]

"The quest for a fit, fat-free body has become an American obsession," Roberta Pollack Seid perceptively points out in *Never Too Thin: Why Women Are at War with Their Bodies*. She adds:

Most Americans probably cannot remember a time when being overweight was not a problem. But in recent years, concern about it has both intensified and spread. Barely a decade ago we strove for thinness and health. Today, swept up by the "wellness epidemic," we pant for fitness and super-health. This shift in emphasis has not changed our underlying goal—a fat-free body—but it has made that goal more complex, paramount and insidious. It has also expanded the ranks of fat fighters. . . .

The modest prescription, "Watch your weight, eat right, and exercise" has become a national compulsion and a national creed. The obsession has spawned a multibillion-dollar, recession-proof industry that continues to expand yearly, and it has infiltrated countless other industries. It has triggered an upheaval in America's life-style and affects our social relationships, our festivities, and our leisure activities. It has altered our attitudes about our bodies and has seduced us into letting these body attitudes profoundly affect both our judgments about our characters and our emotional and psychological reality. It is a compulsion that has totally disrupted that private and formerly very pleasurable necessity—eating.[3]

Three out of every four Americans are actively engaged—physically and/or mentally—in this struggle each day. Consequently, many of us no longer eat normally due to the food deprivation we've endured for the sake of losing weight.

It isn't only adults who experience this inner turmoil: recent studies suggest that 50 to 80 percent of fourth-grade girls have already started dieting.[4] When interviewed by a reporter from *The Wall Street Journal,* two of the girls who participated in one of these studies said, "Boys expect girls to be beautiful and perfect, and skinny," and "Fat girls aren't like regular girls—they aren't attractive."

According to the *American Journal of Diseases of Children,*

12 percent of junior and senior-high school girls diet at least 10 times a year. Also, juvenile dieters tend to experience the same unhealthy consequences of habitual starvation as their older counterparts: they're more likely to suffer from a poor body image, eating binges, and fears that they can't stop eating. They're also more likely to use self-induced vomiting, laxatives, and diuretics to lose weight.[5]

Self-Hating Beauty Behaviors

One of the most devastating results of our cultural outlook on food is that each year, approximately one million women develop anorexia nervosa or bulimia, debilitating eating disorders that are classified as unique forms of mental illness.[6] While anorexia and bulimia are treatable if women obtain help soon enough, both disorders are also potentially fatal.

The American Anorexia and Bulimia Association (AA/BA) reports that 150,000 women die of anorexia nervosa in the United States every year. It's now estimated that at least 20 percent of American college women regularly binge and purge.[7]

Years ago, while working as an assistant to a professor of family wellness at the University of Nebraska, I began to question cultural attitudes and assumptions about weight control. Having bounced from dieting to overeating countless times, my own defenses against fat were fairly heavily fortified, reinforced by the weight loss regimens I'd followed over a dozen years. But when I came face-to-face with the life-threatening eating disorders of students who came to me, I began to see dieting much differently.

One of my responsibilities was to check the student's body-fat percentages with electronic calipers—measuring the skin-fold widths overlying muscle tissue at certain key places on the body. I also ran computerized "diet checks" to evaluate each student's total nutritional intake over a three-day period. Over six consecutive terms, I noticed that about one out of every five female students fit a classic eating-disorder profile: all were high achievers—many were also sorority members—with body-fat percentages of less than 15 percent, and total nutritional intakes of under 800 calories daily.

Lists of foods eaten usually consisted of diet soft drinks throughout the day, a candy bar for breakfast, lettuce salad without dressing for lunch, and a slice of pizza or a McDonald's hamburger with perhaps a few French fries for dinner, if an evening meal was eaten at all. A late night snack of plain popcorn or an apple might be indulged in a couple of times per week, but that was all. Several of the students ate far less than 800 calories per day. A couple had only orange juice for breakfast. Some avoided meat and sugar altogether. None ate anything close to what could be called a balanced diet—one that supplied their Recommended Daily Allowance of vitamins or involved eating foods from the Food Pyramid every day.

In addition to noticing these highly malnutritive eating practices, I also observed that the students had extensive, elaborate exercise regimens and were highly praised for doing so: they were among the most popular women at school and were greatly rewarded for their fine, svelte figures. Fine as in thin. Amazingly thin! The ultimate in thinness.

They were so thin, in fact, that many of the affected women had stopped menstruating and constantly complained of being cold. I also noticed they never liked to sit very long in hard wooden chairs because their pelvic bones were no longer sufficiently padded to do so.

I quickly became concerned—and angered—as I observed the isolated one-woman hunger camps these students had locked themselves into. Literally starving to be beautiful, they disguised their gaunt appearance, thinning hair, and bony legs so it wouldn't bother anybody. In fact, these women were noticed precisely because they had successfully managed to punish their bodies into unnatural thinness in their all-out war against fat. I couldn't help wondering: what if this same amount of thought and energy were being directed toward something really life-changing and worthwhile instead?

When I mentioned my concerns to these women, handing out referrals to an eating disorders program on campus, they'd simply smile and look at me as if *I* were the one who was sick.

Telling students that a body-fat percentage of 25 to 30 percent is perfectly healthy and normal for a woman—when they were completely convinced that any fat at all was disgustingly ugly—somehow seemed useless when every air-brushed advertisement, popular women's magazine, and successful celebrity's portrait portrays beauty as never being larger than a size seven.

How else can we expect young women to respond?

Chronic Dieting and Anorexia: Religious Roots

Chronic dieting, self-starvation, and anorexia nervosa aren't new—they're just more prevalent today, and are occurring for a wider variety of reasons. If we think it's only American culture that has trapped women into equating thinness with self-mastery, we need to think again. In medieval Europe more than 700 years ago, refusal of food and prolonged fasting were considered desirable goals and an exclusively female miracle among Christian women.[8]

Numerous historical records of women saints who lived between A.D. 1200-1500 verify that many ate almost nothing or strictly limited their diets by claiming to actually be unable to eat food that felt satisfying to their flesh. When cultural beliefs about thinness link up to the denial of food for spiritual reasons, life-threatening eating disorders can result.

Catherine of Siena (A.D. 1347-1380), for example, consumed only a handful of herbs every day, and sometimes even shoved twigs down her throat to purge herself after being forced to eat nutritious food. Mary of Oignes and Beatrice of Nazareth, who lived during the thirteenth century, vomited if they caught a whiff of meat, their throats often swelling in the mere presence of food. Some women saints covered their faces at the sight of food, and at least one—Columba of Rieti in the fifteenth century—actually perished as a result of refusing to eat. In the seventeenth century, Saint Veronica regularly fasted for three days at a time and, on Fridays, permitted herself to chew only on five orange seeds while meditating on the five wounds of

Christ.[9] (In contrast to these historical accounts, apparently very few male saints claimed to be incapable of eating.)

For these women, fasting was an essential component to feminine holiness, a fantastic form of proof they could survive without food by partaking in prayer and Holy Communion instead. Survivors of this rigid form of Christian asceticism, later termed *anorexia mirablis* ("miraculously inspired loss of appetite"), became widespread from the thirteenth to fifteenth centuries.

Medieval culture promoted this deadly form of appetite control through its belief that the female body itself is integrally associated with food. As a result, pious women became preoccupied with denying the earthly pleasures of food and its power over them. Eating and fasting provided an especially effective means of denying the shame associated with their sexuality, as well as giving them a unique way to express their religious ideals through bodily suffering.[10]

Of the 261 Italian holy women who have lived over the last eight centuries—those officially recognized by the Roman Catholic Church as saints, blesseds, venerables, or servants of God—more than half displayed clear signs of anorexia, which is defined as the loss of appetite or aversion to food.[11]

In Ecclesiastes 2:24-25, Solomon says, "A man can do nothing better than to eat and drink and find satisfaction in his work. This too, I see, is from the hand of God, for without him, who can eat or find enjoyment?" Nothing could be stated more plainly than this: the Bible calls eating a gift of God![12] Furthermore, the Kingdom of God doesn't have anything to do with what we eat (or don't eat)—it's a matter of freely receiving God's good gifts of righteousness, peace, and joy in the Holy Spirit.[13]

As many of the medieval saints did, Christian women today are also increasingly equating austere eating and exercising with obedience to God. Because of the culture in which we live and the intimate connection between eating behaviors and ideals of self-control, we're particularly vulnerable to developing eating disorders as Christian women in our culture.

Fasting and self-control are Christian disciplines that play an important role in our walk with God, to be sure, but Scripture clearly calls us to care for our bodies—not abuse them. For a woman struggling with an eating disorder, any form of fasting is best avoided until underlying emotional needs are confronted and resolved.

*Dieting Is **Not** the Solution*

As individuals, our self-image will automatically reflect and represent the collective culture in which we live, unless we stand back and critically examine that culture, then commit ourselves to making a change. A sociologist accomplishes this, to some degree, through intensive research and classroom instruction. A feminist might do the same thing through weekly "consciousness-raising" sessions. A psychotherapist attempts to alter a person's self-perceptions through guided discussion and focused introspection.

Christians, however, can wisely combine the truth of Scripture and comprehensive Bible study, prayer, the infilling and guidance of the Holy Spirit, and an ongoing reciprocal relationship with a local body of believers to gain an accurate picture of how our identities have been warped by our culture and distorted the way we see ourselves. Like other women, we can easily fall prey to forming a self-image based on cultural and church-related stereotypes rather than on the Word of God. Perhaps more than any other dimension of our identity, bondage to weight-based beauty ideals can grip our minds and distort our thinking. We can easily get sucked into this worldly perspective on food and fat unless we ask the Lord to free us.

Today's weight-loss industry teaches a doctrine of dieting that falsely promises women everything from greater financial freedom to romantic success—and makes dieting itself into a near-religion. In the Bible, Christians are called to resist conforming to this kind of mold.

According to biologist Dr. Dale M. Artens, we shouldn't find this surprising. That's because the belief systems that diet doctrines teach aren't based on reality but on a magical way of thinking. He asserts:

> Fat, in most cases, is not a health hazard, and weight loss is not a generally desirable ideal. . . . The view that all fat is ugly is an unnatural and unhealthy prejudice. Nor is it simply a matter of choosing to be fat or thin. Fatness and thinness are reflections of fundamental physiological processes over which we have surprisingly little control. Dieting and exercise have remarkably short-term effects on body weight.
>
> The international religious community of dieters is bound together by an uncommonly small creed. Fat is evil. Slenderness is salvation. The diet messiahs paint apocalyptic visions of doom visited upon those who refuse to purge themselves of the sin of fat. They paint visions of fulfillment and of the full bounty of social largesse visited upon those who choose to be saved. Beauty, love, and longevity are all there, simply awaiting your embrace.[14]

"Dieting has become a religion," claims Los Angeles psychologist Dr. Nancy Bonus. "It's no longer about health; it's about morality. If you gain weight you're a bad person; if you lose weight you're a good person. We have a religion-like shrine in our bathroom—the scale—and when you step on that hunk of metal it determines your value as a person." [15]

In a recent interview, the founder of Weight Watchers, Jean Nidetch, admits: "I like a cookie. Sometimes two. That's sinful for me." [16] Since founding the organization 30 years ago, 25 million members in twenty-four countries have heard the goodness and badness of food preached about through the Weight Watchers gospel. While their promotion of healthy lifestyles is commendable, equating eating a couple of cookies with breaking God's law is going too far. When Nidetch says, "If you can lose weight, you can do anything," it's instantly apparent she's making a serious sales pitch—not citing a scientifically based claim about eating behavior.[17]

No data can back up weight-loss program claims that you will lose weight and not gain it back. In fact, most obesity experts now agree that just the opposite is true. When a National Institute of Health panel convened to discuss the topic in 1992, it concluded that the vast majority of people who diet will, sooner or later, put the weight back on. In the few studies that have examined the long-term impact of commercial weight-loss regimens, it's been shown that more than 90 percent of dieters who lost 25 pounds gain the weight back within two years.[18]

A recent study published in *Consumer Reports* confirms this research. After conducting the first large-scale survey of the major diet programs, *CR* found that "despite their sales pitches, there is no evidence that commercial weight-loss programs help most people achieve significant, permanent weight loss."[19] Basing their findings on information gleaned from some 95,000 readers, *CR* discovered that, although people initially lose weight, the great majority gain it back within two years.

> If you want or need to lose weight, you would probably do well to try to reduce on your own, or through a free hospital-based program, before spending money on a commercial weight loss center. . . . Most important, given the strong likelihood that any weight lost on a reducing diet will be gained back promptly, we recommend that anyone contemplating a diet think seriously about whether losing weight is necessary or desirable in the first place. As our survey and others have shown, many people diet even though they are not overweight. . . . the majority of dieters would probably do better to forget about cutting calories, focus on exercising and eating a healthful diet, and let the pounds fall where they may.[20]

"It is the taking off and the putting on of weight that endangers the body," says Dr. Hillel Schwartz in his book, *Never Satisfied.* "No one has been able to prove that fatness *per se* cuts life short. If left alone, 99 percent of human beings will reach a plateau weight, a set point at which their metabolisms will be satisfied and their bodies healthy. It is the dieting, the anxiety, and the perpetual scrimmaging with food that lead to illness."[21]

Time for a Change

Of 33,000 women polled by *Glamour* magazine, fully 75 percent between the ages of 18 and 35 believed themselves to be too fat. Only 25 percent of the women surveyed were overweight by medical standards, and of those who were underweight, 45 percent still thought they were too heavy. Respondents also said that they would rather lose 10 to15 pounds than achieve any other goal.[22]

How many Christians have fallen into this trap? I think many of us have, simply by virtue of being contemporary American women. Unless we make a concerted effort to change this way of thinking, it's pretty much guaranteed: we *will* become chronic dieters, worry about our weight, and view the body weight of others critically.

Dr. Kathy Bowen-Woodward, a specialist on eating disorders, explains part of the reason why this happens to so many women today:

> When we look at the models in the magazines or the women on TV to see whether we are thin enough, we forget that these models are "abnormally" built. Their figures do not generally occur in nature. They work very hard to develop their bodies, and they have to work constantly to maintain what they have created. For every model we see in a magazine, there are many who were turned away because they were too tall or too heavy or just didn't have the right "look." This means that when we look at a model, we're looking at the rare exception rather than the general rule. We're seeing what you can be if you have just the right ingredients to begin with, if you work unceasingly to bring your body within certain limits, if you are continually preoccupied with your body, if you have a team of professionals doing your wardrobe, and if you are very lucky. Yet most of us don't think about that when we look at newspapers or magazines. We think we're looking to see how we're supposed to look. We think we're just making sure we're OK.
>
> And we decide we're not. So we start to diet and exercise and skip meals and do all the things we think will let us

look like the models, and if only we can look like them we'll be OK. But since few of us can look like them, most of us end up on a cycle that goes nowhere but leaves us chronically dissatisfied and preoccupied with our bodies. [23]

To better assess how our own attitudes have been affected in this area, the following 20 questions enable us to understand the extent of our participation in today's diet culture.[24]

Food Attitudes:
A Personal Assessment

1. Do I think about food at other times than when I'm hungry?
   Yes ___ No ___

2. Do I often notice what other people eat—and how much and how often they eat?
   Yes ___ No ___

3. Do I respond to hunger by eating enough to satisfy me and nourish my body, or by overeating (or undereating)?
   Yes ___ No ___

4. Do I eat only when I'm hungry and stop when I'm not?
   Yes ___ No ___

5. Do I worry or often think about my weight?
   Yes ___ No ___

6. Do I frequently worry about what I eat and feel angry or disgusted with myself if I eat too much?
   Yes ___ No ___

7. Do I continually count calories (or fat grams or carbohydrates or whatever the latest fad dictates)?
   Yes ___ No ___

8. Do I diet—avoid certain types of foods for the purpose of losing

weight or not gaining weight—frequently?
Yes ___ No ___

9. Do I look at magazines, TV ads, or exercise videos and think the models appear to be of "normal" weight?
Yes ___ No ___

10. Do I ever use laxatives or make myself vomit after eating too much?
Yes ___ No ___

11. Do I sometimes avoid going out if I feel fat?
Yes ___ No ___

12. Do I criticize others for their eating habits, whether silently or out loud?
Yes ___ No ___

13. Do I feel like my day is ruined if I've gained weight or have eaten too much?
Yes ___ No ___

14. Do I find that staying hungry gives me a feeling of being in control?
Yes ___ No ___

15. Do I usually notice what size people are before I notice other things about them?
Yes ___ No ___

16. Do I ever feel ashamed about the size of my body?
Yes ___ No ___

17. Do I see women with the kind of body I'd like to have and wish I could look like them?
Yes ___ No ___

18. Do I weigh myself more often than once or twice a month?
Yes ___ No ___

19. Do I exercise for any reason other than I enjoy it and it makes me feel better—and if I happen to miss exercising, does it make me feel fat?
Yes ___ No ___

20. Do I feel disgusted or ashamed with myself when I feel fat and proud of myself when I feel thin?
Yes ___ No ___

Answering yes to more than three or four of these questions indicates you have an unrealistic perception of your body—a distorted body image; more than five means you're also at risk for acquiring an eating disorder. If you identified with more than 10 of these questions, you don't need a new diet or exercise routine—you need a complete change from the inside out.[25]

There aren't many of us who can read through these questions and answer no to every single one. I can't. As a matter of fact, there are lots of us who can answer yes to almost *all* of them.

I like what writer Laura Fraser has learned as a result of a lifetime of fighting fat. Commenting that she has been obsessed over her body size since she was "a chubby child who practiced arithmetic by counting calories," she adds:

> I first joined Weight Watchers at the age of twelve, lining up to be weighed with women who wore flimsy summer dresses in the dead of winter. There I learned "good" foods and "bad" foods and knew that when I went off my diet, I too was bad. And I was very bad: I yo-yo-dieted all through high school, down and up to 175 pounds, until finally one diet spun out of control into a serious eating disorder.
>
> That was fifteen years ago. Since then I've slowly regained my equilibrium, eating whatever I like (mainly healthy, low-fat foods, it turns out), taking great pleasure in exercising, and rarely weighing myself. I'm strong and sturdy and have no weight problems that can't be nicely solved with a gathered skirt or palazzo pants. It happens that my approach fits the current scientific wisdom, which holds that diets rarely work

long-term, that quick weight loss is dangerous, and that the best way to lose weight is to exercise more rather than eat less, choosing low-fat foods and learning to be comfortable with a body type that may not be exactly svelte.[26]

A score of diet-disabled celebrities including Oprah Winfrey, Delta Burke, and Tracey Gold echo Fraser's refrain. Within months after towing a little red wagon filled with animal fat onto the set of her show, it quickly became apparent that Oprah's 67 pound weight loss had only been temporary. Declaring her Optifast diet a failure, Oprah announced, "I'll Never Diet Again!" on the cover of *People* magazine. She further explained:

> I've been dieting since 1977, and the reason I failed is that diets don't work. I tell people, if you're underweight, go on a diet and you'll gain everything you lost plus more. Now I'm trying to find a way to live in a world with food without being controlled by it, without being a compulsive eater. That's why I say I will never diet again. . . . What is the issue is getting healthy, getting fit and being strong.[27]

Delta Burke, who was slim in early episodes of "Designing Women," slowly added weight with each passing season. Culminating in an abrupt gain of forty pounds, the actress used the change to advantage in one of the series' best shows, titled "They Shoot Fat Women, Don't They?" Delta received her first Emmy nomination for the part. Today, she refuses to abuse her body with dieting, and has switched to a healthier, physiologically sound approach to weight reduction. "I'm not in a race with myself," she says. "The body is a miraculous thing; it knows more than we think it does."[28]

When a diet company recently offered her one million dollars to use and endorse its products, Delta firmly refused. "If I became a spokesperson for a diet product, I'd be saying. . . that unless you're thin, you're not worthwhile," she points out. "When I was in my twenties, I went on a lot of terrible diets. I'd fallen for society's dictates on the way you're supposed to look. I didn't think I was pretty enough or good enough as I was—and I did myself a lot of damage." [29]

For Tracey Gold, a star of ABC's former show "Growing Pains," dieting as a way of life nearly resulted in death. Her downward spiral started after she, then 133 pounds, was told by a doctor that her ideal weight was 113. "He put me on a 500-calorie-a-day diet, and he taught me how to basically starve myself, even knowing I had a past history of anorexia," shares Tracey. But after reaching her goal in just two months, the daily dieting continued.[30]

When the scales eventually dipped down to 90 pounds, Tracey chose hospitalization instead of starvation. Like Oprah and Delta, she acknowledges that the road back to health takes time. "They've stabilized my weight now," she says, "and I'm healthy enough to know that I don't want to lose any more."[31]

Why We Aren't What We Eat

The purpose of this chapter isn't to make ourselves feel worse about eating than we already do or to suggest a comprehensive, individualized treatment plan if we're suffering from an eating disorder, or negative body-image. Instead, the main message is that *we're living in an era that has vaulted beauty ideals to the level of idolatry, and consequently, many of us are trapped by today's beauty culture without exactly knowing how or why or what we can do about it.* This book is my determined attempt to issue a call for freedom through the Lord Jesus Christ, who accepts us just as we are, no matter what we happen to weigh— whether it's 105 or 305 pounds.

We can experience greater freedom regarding eating and what we weigh. While understanding how our culture, family, and genes have shaped our self-concept, we can also receive the healing we need to grow beyond our hurts.

For me, this means that if I suddenly look down at the roll of fat lying over my lower abdomen and it threatens to upset my evening or my love life, I'm allowing something precious to be stolen from me: time, and my joy in being a redeemed participant in the kingdom of heaven.

If I go hungry at the expense of my health, I increasingly realize that I'm choosing to offer myself as a living sacrifice to my culture rather than to the Lord. When I complain about gaining an extra 10 pounds and then dwell upon it, I realize I'm wasting valuable time and energy that would pay eternal dividends if I invested it for God's glory instead.

I'm discovering that I'm not what I eat. Not at all! Jesus frees me from feeling pride and a sense of moral superiority when I'm thinner, and self-conscious shame when I'm heavier—as well as keeping me from judging others based on what they eat or how thin or heavy *they* are.[32]

As I wake up to the grace of God and His goodness toward me, I begin to see all my weaknesses and vulnerabilities in a new light: the light of Christ's unconditional love and the power of His healing salvation. His gentle touch washes away my preoccupation with my looks and the looks of others.

I can see where I want to go, even though my final destination still lies in the distance: "Not that I have already obtained all this, or have already been made perfect, but I press on to take hold of that for which Christ Jesus took hold of me." [33] Most importantly, perhaps, I know the place where I'm headed—and when I get there, I seriously doubt that anyone's going to notice my dress size, my cellulite, or my double chin.

Action Plan

Food For Thought

Information on diet is readily available, but it doesn't hurt to remember that there's hope for habitual dieters and overeaters—two closely connected patterns which many of my friends and I have pondered endlessly over Diet Cokes and chocolate chip cookies.

E. C. Wayne Callaway, an obesity researcher at George Washington University, suggests following these up-to-the-minute guidelines on weight loss. First, learn proper eating habits and eat that way throughout your life to maintain an appropriate weight. Second, exercise regularly. And third, consider working with the emotional causes of overeating.

To lose weight, Dr. Callaway suggests following these guidelines, plus cutting out a couple hundred calories a day from one's diet—the equivalent of a bowl of cereal with milk or a candy bar. It's a far cry from the 800 to 1,000 calorie-a-day counts commonly found in commercial weight-loss programs. Callaway claims that even diets that include as many as 1,200 calories don't work. Those with fewer than 800 are downright dangerous, and all too often result in gallstones, heart disorders, fainting, fatigue, hair loss, headaches, cold intolerance, muscle weakness and cramping, loss of lean tissue, and decreased sexual desire. The human body needs a certain amount of fat and salt to work right; without it, vital systems fail to function properly.

Stating that obesity is caused by a number of complex factors, including genetics, hormones, physical activity, energy output, behaviors, and emotions, Dr. Callaway cautions, "You should never go through a deprivation phase when attempting to lose weight."[34] It may be very difficult for chronic dieters to give up the idea that the way to lose weight is to deprive the body of food and to go on periodic fasts. Regular, healthy eating and enjoyable exercise don't come naturally to someone who has spent years counting calories, calculating food portions, and considering fat grams.

Strategies That May Help:

Resolve to learn more about food and fat facts.

Recent studies show that an enzyme called lipoprotein lipase (LPL) moves fat out of the bloodstream into fat cells for later use. By acting as a highly specialized transportation system, LPL responds to food deprivation in as little as four hours. In summary, what this means is that when given too few calories, the body quickly responds by burning less fat (at least when a person isn't sleeping); upon a return to normal calorie levels, it then stores fat more efficiently.[35]

"Our bodies have tremendously elegant mechanisms

for surviving a famine," Dr. Callaway explains.[36] Knowing this can be an excellent antidote to self-imposed starvation.

Discount confusion and condemnation.

Myths about weight control abound. In most cases, only books written by registered dietitians or doctors, with additional training in the physiology of obesity, offer sound advice. Read these and ignore the rest. Confront any distorted fears and attitudes you've picked up over the years and toss the entire folder out of your memory files. In its place, ask God to give you wisdom and compassion concerning your body and the bodies of others. Notice how overweight people are treated in our society and choose not to act that way. Above all, develop and maintain the ability to laugh about your weight and eating-related issues.

Eat smaller meals throughout the day.

Besides boosting mental alertness and energizing fat metabolism, nibbling is fun. According to one study in the *New England Journal of Medicine*, those who ate 17 (!) small snacks per day fared better than those who ate three large meals.[37] Their conclusion: it isn't only the amount and type of food we eat, but the *frequency* of eating, that contributes to our body weight. Avoiding a starvation mode appears vital in staving off the body's automatic adaptability to famine through sluggish fat-burning and hastened lipid storage. Here are some suggestions:

- Half a toasted bagel with fat-free soft cream cheese
- A fruit salad of chopped bananas, apples, grapes, oranges, melons, and berries tossed with lime juice

and a little honey
- Grape-nuts and vanilla yogurt
- Baked potato (zapped in the microwave several minutes) topped with bacon-bits, chives, salsa, chopped broccoli, shredded mozzarella cheese, low-fat sour cream or ranch-style dressing, etc.
- Apricot halves and cottage cheese
- Low-fat milk blended until frothy with one-quarter cup of berries or half a banana, a dash of spice (cinnamon or nutmeg), and vanilla, sweetened to taste
- Tuna or chicken salad on crackers or melba toast
- Instant pudding, tapioca, or custard made with low fat milk
- Refried beans spread on fresh tortilla triangles, sprinkled with salsa, shredded low-fat cheese, and seasonings, then heated until cheese melts
- Tablespoon of peanut butter on a slice of light whole-wheat bread with a glass of one-percent milk or calcium-enriched orange juice
- Two ounces cranberry juice mixed with eight ounces sparkling water in a tall glass with ice and lemon slices
- Graham crackers with all-fruit raspberry preserves or lemon curd (a spreadable English concoction that reminds me of extra-thick lemon pie filling)
- Mozzarella sticks and peeled baby carrots
- Slice of angel food cake with strawberry jam and whipped topping
- Pita bread stuffed with leaf lettuce, tomato, green pepper, shaved turkey, and thinly sliced provolone
- Apple slices and sugar-free coffee or fruit-flavored yogurt

Be as consistent as possible.

Since bingeing one day and fasting the next can significantly impair one's fat-burning capacity, avoid big ups and downs. In other words, go for a fairly consistent number of calories each day. If the holidays or a special celebration find you zooming way over the top, don't automatically starve yourself the next day—just eat lighter foods, snack frequently, and go for a walk.

Eat when you're hungry; stop when you're not.

This may sound silly, but for me, it was an entirely new concept when I tried it. After years of chronic dieting, I'd learned to ignore my body's signals and use my head to determine what and when to eat instead. My nutritionist was especially helpful in this regard: she held up her hand, made a tight fist, and said, "This is how much food your stomach can hold and digest comfortably." I haven't forgotten her vivid example.

It's been absolutely amazing to give up twice-daily weigh-ins in exchange for a common sense—even childlike—approach to eating. Since adopting this outlook toward eating in 1990, my weight has fluctuated very little. Though I rarely lose weight, I don't often gain it, either—a noteworthy change for me. And, to my relief, I'm now less encumbered by mental lists of "good" and "bad" foods, weight charts, and harsh self-talk.

Reward yourself with things other than food.

This is a biggie for a lot of us, believe me. Whether it's a Dairy Queen ice cream cone or a warm cup of hot chocolate with whipped cream, food soothes us. Consequently, we need to replace some of these gastronomic treats with other emotionally satisfying rewards when we want to be nurtured.

My own list includes reading a good book, digging in my herb garden, listening to music, taking a long, hot bath, and walking briskly under a bright blue sky. I've found that taking time out three or four times daily to recover joy is a smart way to foil food fixations. What do you regularly do for yourself to lighten life's load?

If the "out of control" feeling is too overwhelming to manage on your own, it's entirely appropriate to consult a nutritionist or obtain other support. Don't be afraid of what others will think. If you're concerned about your attitude toward food, get the help you need. Make peace with your body and take courage: how you feel today doesn't have to be the way you feel for the rest of your life.

Exercise often and get enough rest.

Besides deactivating LPL, moderate aerobic exercise performed for a minimum of 30 minutes at least three to four times a week, conditions the heart and promotes the secretion of powerful substances called endorphins, an aid to pain reduction, relaxation, and mood stability.

Forget about going for the burn: engage only in activities you enjoy and feel comfortable doing. If you're currently involved in a personal exercise program, great; if not, it only takes six weeks to experience the benefits of aerobic conditioning. With the wide range of choices available today, there's truly something for people of every shape, size, and stage of life.

In addition to aerobic activity, your body will also benefit from getting the rest it requires. By paying attention to fatigue and food cues, you may find that you're less likely to overeat, use hunger to keep you going, or use food to meet your emotional needs. Don't be surprised if you need more than seven or eight hours nightly, plus a brief snooze or quiet time sometime during the day: doze on demand and see if it helps.

❧ *Focus Questions* ❧

1. To what extent has your dress size determined your attitude about your body? Do you fear wearing a larger size (say, size 10 compared to size six, or size 16 instead of size 12)? If so, why?

2. Over the years, you may have acquired a poor body image or an eating disorder—most likely as a result of living in a fat-phobic society and/or family. How has the fear of fat affected your life most? How does this fit with what the Bible says about who you are in Christ?

3. What are 10 reasons why your weight is not the most important thing in your life on which to be concentrating your time, energy, and attention?

❧ *Five* ❧

Beauty By Knife

Sure. Why not do it? You have body work done
on your car.
—— *Sylvester Stallone,* People Weekly, *1992*

Beauty stands
In the admiration of weak minds
Led captive.
—— *John Milton,* Paradise Regained, II, *1671*

I recently picked up a free copy of an Atlanta weekly arts and entertainment guide. Inside, a colorful page caught my eye. Across the top, bold letters spelled the words: Video Imaging & Plastic Surgery.

In the photo underneath, a woman with glossy blonde hair, big brown eyes, and a medium-sized nose is shown gazing at an imaginary reflection of herself: on the left side of the picture, she is staring off to the right; on the right, she is looking back toward herself on the left. The two sides are almost identical, with one exception—the woman's picture on the right has a slightly smaller, perkier nose.

The caption beneath the photograph explains why the two images are similar, yet different. It reads: Computer-Simulated Surgical Plan.

A second woman pictured in the ad also models her profile next to one generated by computer. Pictured on the left with a receding chin and prominent, plain-looking nose, the video-enhanced image on the right demonstrates how "improved" the woman's appearance might be if she had both a chin implant and a nose job.

The technological transformation in both cases is remarkable, turning both women into idealized, disembodied shadows of their natural selves. The appealing display makes us wonder how we might be re-designed by such techniques—and once our curiosity is aroused, a free appointment is a phone call away.

"Successful cosmetic surgery," the ad copy beckons, "is achieved by a skilled plastic surgeon and realistic patient goals. Video imaging demonstrates your appearance 'before' and anticipated results 'after.' Call for a complimentary imaging consultation."

Reading the ad, I thought of the unspoken messages conveyed by the pictures—some humorous, some not. For example, if ordinary-looking women (like me) are having this done, I can, too. My big nose (or ears or breasts or mouth) is unattractive, so I'll just change it. It's well worth the time, expense, and pain to have plastic surgery done when I can look so much better, even if it does cost $4,000. Why feel crummy about being a 6.4 on a scale from 1-10, when I could be a 7 or an 8?

What an ad like this doesn't tell us, though, are the less appealing aspects of surgically altering one's body for cosmetic purposes: the pain we'll suffer, the thousands of dollars we'll spend, or the identity shift we'll encounter afterwards. Furthermore, it doesn't say that if we run into complications—which at least 15 percent of all plastic surgery patients do—that we might have to be re-hospitalized and operated on again to remove scar tissue, treat blood clotting, or correct a "poor surgical result." And it also doesn't warn us that we could actually look worse after surgery due to extensive scarring, a botched nose job, or the displacement of an artificial implant.

Most of all, this ad ignores the fact that we're *each totally unique individuals*—one of a kind in the entire universe!—and that it is our royal birthright to celebrate and appreciate our God-given quirks and qualities.

An Operable Condition

Why would we let anyone sculpt us according to some sort of ready-made, prepackaged, computer-created design? Why are so many women submissively sacrificing their natural design to surgeons' scalpels? Is the lust for beauty really so strong in us? Are we that afraid of aging?

Although I disagree with her ideology, I find the observations of Naomi Wolf, author of *The Beauty Myth: How Images of Beauty Are Used Against Women,* to be wonderfully clear on this topic. Taken from a Christian point of view, her vividly poignant remarks are especially illuminating:

> Whatever is deeply, essentially female—the life in a woman's expression, the feel of her flesh, the shape of her breasts, the transformations after childbirth of her skin—is being reclassified as ugly, and ugliness as disease. . . . You could see the signs of female aging as disease, especially if you had a vested interest in making women, too, see them your way. Or you could see that if a woman is healthy she lives to grow old; as she thrives, she reacts and speaks and shows emotion, and grows into her face. Lines trace her thoughts and radiate from the corners of her eyes after decades of laughter, closing together like fans as she smiles. You could call the lines a network of "serious lesions," or you could see that in a precise calligraphy, thought has etched marks of concentration between her brows, and drawn across her forehead the horizontal creases of surprise, delight, compassion, and good talk. A lifetime of kissing, of speaking and weeping, shows expressively around her mouth scored like a leaf in motion. The skin loosens on her face and throat, giving her features a setting of sensual dignity; her features grow stronger as she does. She has looked around in her life, and it shows. . . . The maturing of a woman who has continued to grow is a beautiful thing to behold. Or, if your ad revenue or your seven-figure salary or your privileged sexual status depend on it, it is an operable condition.[1]

Welcome to the brave new world of beauty, brought to you courtesy of your local cosmetic surgeon—a fully licensed and accredited M.D. who makes $200,000 or more annually by treating patients' less-than-perfect appearances as if they were disfiguring disorders.

In the early years of plastic surgery, the few who could afford it—Marilyn Monroe, Milton Berle, and Elvis Presley, for example—tended to be rich, famous, and/or emotionally unstable. (A 1960 report of cosmetic surgery recipients concluded that one-third had personality trait disturbances, 20 percent were neurotic, and 16 percent were psychotic).[2] Having one's nose or breasts "done" was considered an extreme way of dealing with whatever nature had, or hadn't, supplied at birth. For the average American, having plastic surgery for cosmetic purposes was simply unheard of.

Not any longer. The cosmetic surgery industry now grosses $300 million each year and continues to grow unabated at an annual rate of 10 percent. By 1988, more than two million people had undergone plastic surgery—a number that had tripled over the previous two years (the total up until 1986 was 590,556)—and the annual caseload of American plastic surgeons reached 1.5 million people.[3] Nearly 90 percent of the recipients were women. The following figures reflect this trend:

Growth of Plastic Surgery in the 1980s

	1981	*1989*
Face-lifts:	39,000	75,000
Chin Implants:	9,000	17,000
Eyelid Tucks:	56,000	100,000
Breast Implants:	72,000	100,000

| Liposuction: | 1,000 | 250,000 |
| Nose Alterations: | 51,500 | 95,000 [4] |

A recent survey conducted by a plastic surgery association found that about half of their patients earn less than $25,000 per year, requiring them to take out loans and, at times, even mortgage their homes to pay for elective cosmetic surgery.[5] Since it's obvious that several hundred thousand women haven't won the lottery or inherited sizable sums of money lately, what provoked such a sudden, staggering rise in U.S. plastic surgery rates?

Competing for Dollars

Beginning in 1983, the American Society of Plastic and Reconstructive Surgeons (ASPRS) launched a massive campaign that included a barrage of press releases, "educational" brochures and videos, and carefully screened "before" and "after" photos for physicians' use in local communities. The ASPRS wasn't simply encouraging members to advertise for their share of an already existing market. Instead, the ads were specifically designed to create a new market.

By 1981, cosmetic surgery had become the fastest growing medical specialty in the United States. As the number of plastic surgeons rose—500 percent over two decades—requests for services fell substantially short of the number of physicians who had entered the cosmetic surgery business. This created a supply-and-demand crisis: there were far too many plastic surgeons with much too little to do. (Sadly, and to our shame, this has taken place in a country where millions of Americans still lack health insurance and have trouble obtaining basic health care.)

Faced with this challenging economic dilemma, the ASPRS went after the public's attention, and our wallets, by professionally designing and implementing a nation-wide marketing scheme.[6] Plastic surgeons blitzed the media: in magazines and newspapers, on radio and television, even on local billboards. Popular women's magazines published dozens of stories "selling" readers on the wonders of cosmetic surgery and its career and romance-enhancing capabilities. By pairing supportive articles with attractive ads, a boom industry successfully created its own demand for services.

"Feel more confident about yourself," said one ad for the Center for Aesthetic & Reconstructive Surgery. "Go curvy," *Mademoiselle* suggested on its cover. "Pursue career goals," declared another ad in *The New York Times. Vogue* and *The Wall Street Journal* recommended women should view breast enlargement surgery and fat suctioning as a positive "investment" to further their personal and career goals. Even *Ms.* magazine promoted plastic surgery as a way to strategically "reinvent" one's self, encouraging women to "dare to take control of your life" by having plastic surgery.[7]

The most famous ad to date, carried by *L.A. Magazine*, is an eight-page fold-out featuring a full-breasted woman in a bathing suit alongside a red Ferrari, accompanied by the slogan: "Automobile by Ferrari. Body by Forshan." The ad refers to Dr. Vincent Forshan, a plastic surgeon practicing in Rancho Mirage, California. But as it turns out, Forshan had never even operated on the woman; another physician, Dr. Charles Smithdeal of Los Angeles, had. After arguments about false advertising and resulting disclaimers ensued between the doctors, a later issue of the magazine tried to correct the error. Using exactly the same model and Ferrari, the message simply read: "Body by Smithdeal." [8] Apparently, the old days of plastic surgery are over.

Today, with nearly half the world's plastic surgeons practicing in the United States (one-third are in California), the cosmetic surgery industry has mushroomed into a three-billion-dollar-per-year business.[9]

Signs of the Times

As I was preparing to write this chapter, *People Weekly* devoted an entire cover story on "Plastic Surgery of the Stars," including a "Did They or Didn't They?" photo essay of well-known celebrities and their noteworthy facial changes over the years. "Anyone who has ever splurged on a cruise or a trip to Europe can now save up for self-beautification instead," wrote journalist Marjorie Rosen in the featured article, adding that "for an increasing number of women—and men—cosmetic surgery is an acceptable antidote to the inequity of nature and the cumulative effects of roast beef and gravity." [10]

The list of famous cosmetic surgery recipients appears to be endless, and includes Elizabeth Taylor, Nancy Reagan, Cher, Angela Lansbury, Jane Fonda, Betty Ford, Kenny Rogers, Rosalynn Carter, Bette Midler, Jacqueline Kennedy Onassis, and Phyllis Diller.

Incredibly, Ms. Diller, known as Hollywood's reigning Queen of Plastic Surgery, claims she has spent over $50,000 on having her face lifted (twice), abdomen stitched tighter, teeth straightened and bonded, breasts reduced, nose changed (twice), chin tightened, eyes lifted, cheeks implanted, facial skin chemically peeled, and eyebrows raised in an all-out war against her body's natural appearance.[11]

"Plastic surgery is mandatory for a lot of what makes for successful leading men and ladies," a Beverly Hills plastic surgeon, Dr. George Semel, reminds us. "There are very few who can get by without a little help."[12] Well, apparently more and more Americans are coming to believe that it's not only the rich and famous who need "a little help" these days. The ad campaigns are actually working. Rather than sensibly asking, "Why do women need cosmetic surgery?" people are now wondering, "Why *not?*"

Risks of Cosmetic Surgery

Cosmetic surgery is a sensitive issue. Consequently, if you've had an operation aimed at improving your appearance, it's likely that you tried to make the best possible decision given your conditions and personal circumstances. After all is said and done, each of us needs to evaluate the benefits and risks of a specific procedure when considering plastic surgery.

For women whose self-esteem has been shattered by an accident or illness, reconstructive or cosmetic surgery restores something precious: a sense of being oneself again. Birth-related physical abnormalities, rather than leading to a lifetime of stigma and exclusion, may be eased, or even erased, by a surgeon's skill. *The value of medical treatment in such situations cannot be overestimated.*

But in most cases, people have plastic surgery for purely cosmetic reasons—to alter or improve their normal, natural appearance. It used to be considered weird to seek out a plastic surgeon for the purpose of having one's nose reshaped or breasts enlarged. Now, it isn't just widely accepted, it's almost expected! Not surprisingly, many of us have bought into this way of thinking without prayerfully considering all of the issues involved.

On a television commerial, an attractive woman says, "I don't intend to grow old gracefully." If we were truthful, we'd have to admit that phrase is rattling around in our heads, too, and we'd probably add, right along with her, "I intend to fight it every step of the way." It's difficult *not* to acquire this defiant attitude toward aging in a culture that worships youthful bodies, sleek physiques, and beautiful faces.

Yet, aging isn't a disfiguring disease. God created us and loves us just the way we are—wrinkles, warts, and all—whether we're 14 or 94. If we don't accept ourselves, aren't we putting our opinion above our Creator's? Isn't it really self-centered arrogance to want to trade in our body parts for a better-designed (or younger) model?

Learning to come to terms with this isn't easy in our society. When swimsuit season hits, plastic surgeons' appointment books fill up fast. Nevertheless, we can offer a liberating alternative to those who feel trapped in a body they can't change. Facing our own vulnerability and finding a biblical perspective is essential.

Beyond this, there are plenty of excellent reasons why not to have cosmetic surgery. Surgery isn't like buying makeup or getting one's hair done. We are talking about an operation, complete with risks: infection, blood loss, and other possibilities. Besides the fact that it mutilates our highly individualized uniqueness, it's *expensive, unnecessary,* and it *hurts.* Sure, we might look a little "better" (according to someone's standard) after the swelling subsides, the stitches are out, and the bruising goes away. Then again, we might not.

In 1988, a congressional subcommittee looked into a few of the unadvertised aspects of today's plastic surgery industry. The investigation discovered widespread medical abuse, poorly equipped facilities, major injuries, and even deaths from operations performed by unscrupulous, untrained physicians throughout the country. Some plastic surgeons admitted that up to a quarter of their medical practice was devoted to correcting other surgeons' errors. [13]

Because "there is no standard method used for preoperative screening," Congress learned, most women are considered operable. In addition, 90 percent of cosmetic surgery performed in the United States occurs in unregulated offices.[14]

People who testified blamed the FTC (Federal Trade Commission) for permitting plastic surgeons to run advertisements for their services and then to abandon their responsibility for the damage the surgery caused.

Cosmetic surgery patients, who do find a qualified physician, receive no insurance benefits related to their elective surgery. Thus, any complications that result aren't covered by insurance. Problems requiring extra medical care occur in about 30 out of every 200 cases and can quickly add up to thousands of dollars in extra medical bills. Most women seeking cosmetic surgery today feel "it won't happen to me." But in reality, complications can include:

- Severe bruising, infection, and excessive bleeding, requiring ambulance transport, hospitalization, blood transfusions, additional surgery, prescription-strength painkillers, and/or antibiotic therapy;

- Risks related to anesthesia, including cardiac arrest, stroke, allergic response to anesthesia or medications used, or respiratory distress;

- Abnormal blood clot formation in leg or pelvic veins or a dislodged blood clot from the lungs;

- Upper respiratory problems, including pneumonia and bronchitis;

- Accidental damage to surrounding tissue and body structures, which often requires additional surgery and hospitalization;

- Numbness, facial paralysis, and nerve damage, sometimes necessitating microsurgery and nerve grafting;

- Massive loss of skin requiring skin grafting; bad scarring and adhesions, requiring surgical treatment later on;

- Movement, displacement, extrusion (forcing out through the skin), and hardening of scar tissue related to surgically implanted materials, possibly requiring surgical correction;

- Blindness and other permanently disabling or disfiguring physical injuries; and

- Poor aesthetic results, which may or not be corrected by additional plastic surgery.[15]

Subtle Warnings Increase Sales

Even books promoting plastic surgery clearly point out that all such operations are expensive and carry grave risks—though lists of costs and complications are often buried somewhere deep in the text to minimize potential patients' anxiety.

"In every surgeon's life there are cases with unsatisfactory results," admits reporter John Camp in his book *Plastic Surgery: The Kindest Cut*. "But the general situation—that all physicians have poor outcomes in some cases—is well known."[16] It is so well known, in fact, that there's an entire two-volume, 1,134 page medical reference book called *The Unfortunate Result in Plastic Surgery*, which details how to correct a plastic surgeon's mistakes.

In her manual, *The Complete Book of Cosmetic Surgery*, surgeon Dr. Elizabeth Morgan explains it this way:

> Surgery is not guaranteed. Your result is not mass-produced like a car rolling off an assembly line. Your result is more akin to the work of an artist—and everyone knows that even the great Monet painted some pictures that are better than others. He didn't—and couldn't—guarantee a patron a great work of art. Your surgeon cannot guarantee your result, either.[17]

Later, Dr. Morgan adds, "An utterly unforeseen infection or a nerve lying in an abnormal position can cause a disaster no matter how skilled the surgeon is."[18]

Facing the possibility of failure inherent in all cosmetic operations is daunting to even the most highly skilled surgeons. "If you take out a gallbladder and the wound gets infected and you have a healing problem, well, you manage it. At the end of the road, the patient's gallbladder is out and that's what you started out to do," points out Dr. Bruce Cunningham, a surgeon at the University of Minnesota. "If you take a woman who wants a facelift, and she gets an infection, has problems with healing and winds up with scars, you've done exactly the opposite of what you started to do. You've made things worse, not better."[19]

Cher is a rare celebrity, who openly discusses her cosmetic surgeries. Part of the reason may be her own "unfortunate result." "I've had my breasts done," says the well-known actress and singer. "But my breast operations were a nightmare. They were really botched in every way. If anything, they were worse after than before."[20]

Talk show host Jenny Jones couldn't agree more: since getting her first breast implants in 1981, she's spent $20,000 on four additional sets of the devices and has had five separate surgeries performed.[21] Facing yet another operation, she eventually plans to have the implants removed. Warned of the likely results of removing them—severe scarring, indentations, and numbness—Jones is now after safety, not looks. "The cycle has taken me to where I started," she says. "I started with a bad body image . . . [now] I hate my body, and I can't fix it."[22]

"The best plastic surgeons will go out of their way to explain what you will go through," acknowledges reporter Steven Findlay in a cover story for *U.S. News & World Report*. "But many may not fill you in completely. They avoid emphasizing the negative for fear of scaring you off."[23] The recent dispute over silicone breast implants highlights this problem.

Breast Implants Go Bust

In January 1992, the FDA placed a moratorium on silicone breast implants following months of heated debate, dozens of magazine and newspaper articles, numerous talk show discussions, and a formal congressional hearing.[24] Fearful of lawsuits, the implants' primary manufacturer, the Dow Corning Corporation, declared it no longer planned to make the devices.[25]

What many people still don't know about this controversy is that the temporary ban and later restrictions imposed on silicone breast implants—as well as Dow's decision to cease producing them—didn't take place until almost 10 years after the FDA had issued its first warning concerning their use. [26]

"We've performed an experiment on millions of women with an unproved medical device," claims Dr. Douglas R. Shankin, a University of Tennessee pathologist who studies breast tissue from those who have had implants.[27] Harry Spiera, M.D., chief of rheumatology at New York City's Mount Sinai Medical Center, agrees. "The full impact may not be apparent yet," he says, "because so much time can elapse between implant surgery and onset of symptoms."[28]

Public hearings on breast implants drew testimony from scores of affected women and medical experts. Their concerns included the fact that implants rupture and leak silicone into the body, resulting in a variety of autoimmune diseases such as lupus, rheumatoid arthritis, and scleroderma. They can also interfere with breast cancer detection and cause capsular contracture, in which an envelope of fibrous tissue hardens around the implant. Women with implants also reported experiencing skin rashes, joint pain, chronic fatigue, swollen lymph nodes, fever, burning sensations, mental confusion, and loss of nerve sensitivity in their breasts.

In April 1991, after a congressional subcommittee

responded to this testimony, the FDA gave the makers of implants 90 days to prove the efficacy and safety of their products.[29] When they failed to do this, the government agency put a halt to implant sales nearly nine months later, and in April 1992, it issued a final report which curbed the use of silicone implants for cosmetic reasons and strictly limited their availability to reconstructive breast surgery.[30] During the 10 years that these negotiations between the federal government, chemical companies, plastic surgeons, and concerned consumers dragged on, an estimated 1,000,000 women had the sacs of chemical gel implanted, generating hundreds of millions of dollars in profits for plastic surgeons and implant manufacturers.[31]

Because it's now considered appropriate to try almost anything to improve one's appearance—regardless of the risk of death or permanent disability, more than 100,000 women gambled with their lives and bodies in 1991 to obtain bigger breasts—even after the latest FDA warnings went public. It isn't difficult to understand why: "To 'choose' a procedure that may harden the breasts, result in loss of sensation and introduce a range of serious health problems isn't a choice, it's a scripted response," says writer Laura Shapiro. "Those women who locate their self-esteem in their bra size are accurately reading their culture. Sad to say, they're also surrendering to their culture."[32]

Making Miracles—or Unmaking Medicine?

While some plastic surgery is truly rehabilitative, as in the case of rebuilding a woman's breast following a mastectomy or repairing someone's nose after a car collision, approximately 80 percent of the women seeking plastic surgery today do so solely for cosmetic reasons.[33]

Dr. Robert Harvey, a highly successful plastic surgeon on the West Coast and national spokesman for the Breast Council, describes the difference between reconstructive and plastic surgery this way. While initially attracted to his profession for what he calls "altruistic" reasons (such as working with burn patients), he soon switched to cosmetic procedures, which he rationalizes are "more artistic."

"My wife is forty, but she looks thirty," Dr. Harvey told businessmen at an exclusive luncheon recently. "Eventually, she'll probably want a tummy tuck."[34] As the featured speaker, it was Dr. Harvey's second appearance at San Francisco's all-male Bohemian Club.

What's wrong with this picture? Is this art—or a highly sophisticated form of ritualized body mutilation? (Remember seeing all those tribal women proudly parading their scarred bodies across the pages of *National Geographic*? Before you dismiss this seemingly bizarre comparison too quickly, ponder this: any well-trained anthropologist classifies all surgically accomplished, culturally imposed self-beautifying techniques according to this category of human behavior—regardless of whether a witch doctor or medical doctor does it). Physiological aging, small breasts, and flabby abdomens aren't serious disorders worthy of high-tech surgery.

Beyond the obvious questions we should have about Dr. Harvey's statements, there is another, less obvious, concern: the conflict between today's approach to plastic surgery and traditional medical ethics. Consider, for example, these excerpts from several key texts:

The Lord has imparted knowledge to men, that by their use

of his marvels he may win praise; by using them the doctor relieves pain and from them the pharmacist makes up a mixture (The Apocrypha, *New English Bible*).[35]

Above all, do no harm (The Oath of Hippocrates). [36]

Take heed that ye do not cause a malady to any man; and ye shall not cause any man injury by hastening to cut through flesh and blood with an iron instrument or by branding, but shall observe twice and thrice and only then shall give your counsel. (The Oath of Asaph, a Hebrew physician). [37]

No one has the right to injure his own or anyone else's body except for therapeutic purposes. (Jewish author and ethicist Immanuel Jakobvits).[38]

Do not allow thirst for profit, ambition for renown, and admiration to interfere with my profession, for these are the enemies of truth and love for mankind and they can lead astray in the great task of attending to the welfare of Thy creatures. (Moses Maimonides, *Daily Prayer of the Physician*).[39]

The type of "healing" offered by some physicians today is a far cry from the wise norms that have guarded people's dignity and affirmed the value of human life in previous pagan cultures.

Many of today's plastic surgeons compete for consumer dollars in a highly profitable market. Most are principally engaged in the practice of body sculpturing, not the art of medicine. Such physicians make pain instead of relieving it—primarily by cutting into healthy tissue that isn't diseased in any way. Wielding a knife to make people look better, doctors turn heart monitors, blood pressure sensors, suction tubes, vacuum pumps, I.V.'s, ventilation machines, latex catheters, stainless steel clamps, and sterilized forceps into tools that have nothing to do with healing the body.

Why have doctors warped the healing arts toward slicing and suturing women's *healthy* faces and bodies—and why are women asking them to? Why, even after resorting to plastic surgery, do so many women continue to remain troubled about their appearances, sometimes to the point of going back again and again for more "improvements," to no avail?[40]

Might it partly be because beauty was never a medical problem to begin with, but because it's a holy riddle of God?

Action Plan
Telling Ourselves The Truth

On the list below, place a check next to each surgical procedure you've thought about having—seriously or not. In a separate journal, record your thoughts about why you did or did not go ahead with the operation. (If your reason is because you couldn't afford it, what would you have done if you could?)

—Arm reduction
—Birthmark removal
—Breast enlargement
—Breast reduction
—Brow lift
—Buttock lift
—Chemical peel
—Chin implant
—Chin tuck
—Collagen injections
—Ear reshaping

—Eye lift
—Eye tuck
—Forehead lift
—Hair transplants
—Liposuction
—Lip reduction
—Nose job
—Thigh reshaping
—Tummy tuck
—Other

Read Psalm 139 and write down your personal reflections on what it means to be "fearfully and wonderfully made" by God. Do you believe what the Scripture says? As you pray about your response, which concerns about your body most need the Holy Spirit's touch and a greater measure of God's grace? Commit each specific concern to the Lord. If you've already had cosmetic plastic surgery, this portion of the action plan will be valuable as well.

*& Focus Questions *&*

1. In what ways do our attempts to stay "forever young" prevent us from aging with dignity?

2. If someone offered you the opportunity to have the plastic surgery procedure of your choice performed on you without paying for it, how would you respond?

3. Given the popularity of plastic surgery today, how can Christian women be a witness to the world that the phrase "God doesn't make junk" is an accurate statement?

Six

In Their Image: Woman According to Vogue

Fair Amoret has gone astray;
    Pursue and seek her every lover;
I'll tell the signs by which you may
    The wandering shepherdess discover.

Coquet and coy at once her air,
    Both studied, though both seem neglected;
Careless she is with artful care,
    Affecting to seem unaffected.

With skill her eyes dart every glance,
    Yet change so soon you'd ne'er suspect them;
For she'd persuade they wound by chance,
    Though certain art and aim direct them.

She likes herself, yet others hates
    For that which in herself she prizes;
And, while she laughs at them, forgets
    She is the thing that she despises.

                    William Congreve, Amoret, *1670-1729*

*W*hen Adam and Eve ate from the tree of knowledge, their eyes were opened, they realized they were naked, and the world of fashion was born.

From fig-leaf aprons and animal-skin coats to white linen blouses and designer jeans, a colorful array of clothing design has proliferated over the centuries, distinguishing human beings from all the rest of God's creatures through body adornment and attire. Not only is clothing a prime symbol of culture, gender, social status, and wealth, it's also a paradox: we both *present* ourselves, stylishly clothed so that we look like everyone else, and we *hide* behind the clothing we choose by attempting to blend in with everyone around us. It's been this way ever since the Fall.

While philosophers and journalists may debate the relative "goodness" and "badness" of fashion, clothes are definitely here to stay. They will continue to convey powerful messages about a person's sexuality and income, no matter what opinions arise from the latest round of critics.

Clothing communicates. As Christian women, we need to think about what we're saying through the shape, color, fabric, cost, and design of our body coverings. What are we telling those around us by the clothing we select?

While the old adage, "You can't know a book by its cover," still holds true, wise publishers realize that people are first attracted to a book's cover. This first impression of the book influences the buyer forever after. Smart women know this and make sure the way they dress sends out the right first impression.[1] Obviously, men send out signals through their clothing choices, also, but women currently have a much wider range of socially acceptable possibilities than men do, as well as a more varied repertoire of clothing that carries sexual innuendo.

It isn't wrong to want to look nice, but in a society that equates image with personal success, clothes can easily become the basis of our self-worth. We are better able to rely on Christ for our value if we have examined our attitudes about clothing and have decided to rely less on how we dress and more upon the fact that we are made in God's image. But finding a balance between looking good and finding our true identity in Christ can be challenging, to say the least!

Clothing, unlike book covers, is more often selected by impulse and personal taste (or what happens to be on sale) than by skillful reasoning. Successful merchandisers count on our impulse buying. "It all boils down to giving the consumer something she didn't know she wanted," says sportswear designer Dana Buchman.[2]

But sometimes, the look we end up with isn't what we really want at all. My sister Kerry, who for several years wore lots of leather and Lycra ® spandex, enjoyed the attention she received as a result—until it finally hit her that her clothing was inviting outright sexual harassment. (Although she still defends her right to wear trendy clothing because "it fits well and feels comfortable," she's also growing in her ability to admit that she isn't free to wear anything she wants without considering the impact it has on herself and other people.)

Needless to say, most fashion trends today don't fit the Bible's call for modesty. In fact, the clothing industry has gone so far in the opposite direction, it's easy to miss how our own style-consciousness has been shaped by images that sexualize a woman's appearance and detract from her Christian witness.

Ask any man: the way a woman dresses can signal urban independence, rural responsibility, domestic devotion, or committed careerism—and instantly alerts him to her level of sexual availability, self-protection, sophistication, simplicity, or sleaziness.

I had a golden opportunity to see this truth in action when I spent five days with Kerry on the barrier islands off the coast of southeast Georgia last summer. It was before her change of heart and wardrobe. It would have been pretty humorous if it hadn't been so disheartening.

Throughout our extended Atlantic weekend, I was simultaneously appalled and amazed at people's reactions to my sister. Everywhere we went, guys stared and their girlfriends glared. It was as if Kerry was a magnet with a 100 percent guarantee of drawing forth any lust hanging about her immediate vicinity. While she didn't seem to notice, *I* did. As we walked down the beach to get a frozen yogurt, the responses were remarkable.

It didn't happen only when Kerry was wearing a bikini, it happened all the time, whether we were strolling through a mall, standing in line at a movie theater, or dining in a restaurant. Trust me: it wasn't my sister's statuesque five-feet-nine-inch frame or svelte 110-pound figure that were the primary instigators of this unabashed onslaught—it was her attire. (Can you picture Cindy Crawford or Cher, for example, in a baggy, burnt-orange, polyester pantsuit—without any cosmetics, hairstyle, or jewelry—causing a commotion? No, you can't. But put them in figure-flattering, silk summerwear and ponytails, and they'll turn heads.)

Kerry had abandoned Lycra ® spandex in favor of silk some time ago. The blouses, dresses, and skirts my sister wore on our vacation were right out of the pages of *Vogue* or *Elle* magazines. They were attractively designed, hard-to-find items that couldn't be purchased at regular department stores. Basically, Kerry looked the way a zillion other American women secretly would like to look, *if* they had the body and the money to do so.

Here's what's so ironic: the very "look" the fashion magazines promote, if a person successfully adopts it, wreaks havoc in real life. Maybe that's the point. Women weren't created to look like they do in *Vogue*. Yet how many women feel inwardly dissatisfied when they measure themselves against the latest fashion predictions and fall short of reaching top designers' fantasies? The effect is much like a mirage in the desert. We get a shimmery illusion that promises satisfaction, but has no real substance.

Renoir Versus the Supermodel

We can learn a few fascinating lessons about fashion by visiting one of the nation's leading art museums. Gaze at paintings by Renoir or Rembrandt, then compare pictures of these women to pictures of women on the covers of *Bazaar* and *Cosmopolitan*—the women our culture currently holds forth as aesthetic ideals. What do *you* see?

The most immediate difference we're likely to notice between models in classic paintings and contemporary fashion models is, of course, their size. Who can doubt that the women who posed for Renoir weighed at *least* 160 pounds? These paintings, so revealing in their portrayal of healthy, robust—dare I say *womanly?*—females amidst their everyday surroundings, speak volumes. In comparison, current fashion magazines present a shrunken (albeit shimmery) shadow of what our Creator intends femaleness to be.

In the world of fashion, clothing is used primarily for sexual communication, instead of common sense covering for the body, and the models are there to make it talk. The best models in the business are paid millions to maintain unnatural images of womanhood in order to convey the "right" message through the clothes—a message that's more about erotic fantasy than it is about real women. Of this, *Time* magazine reporter Barbara Rudolph writes:

> Today's pretty women represent a new breed: mannequins with sex appeal, as glamorous as cinema legends, as visible as the designers whose clothes they parade. They earn spectacular loot from their spectacular looks. Because, more than ever, modeling is about money. At a time when spending is down, top mannequins can still make consumers buy, so they are paid millions. The worldwide recession and tough times in the advertising business have made the top models one of the few reliable sales tools. . . .
>
> Some things don't change. Any fresh faced 16-year-old who hopes to blossom into a supermodel must meet certain

minimum requirements. [New York's Elite modeling agency director Monique] Pillard reels them off: she must be at least 5 ft. 9 in., bone thin, have full lips, high cheekbones, large eyes, and a straight, not too prominent nose. Models today are taller and fitter than those of previous generations, with fuller lips and bigger breasts. "The models are still skinny," comments Susan Moncur, 41, a semiretired Paris model, "but with big [breasts]—real or false."

Everyone tells the models they're gorgeous, but as long as they work they must guard against imperfection—the bloodshot eye, the puffy face. They diet rigorously, and smoke to keep weight off. Even on good days, models fret that they are not perfect enough. "A girl comes to a shoot with a pimple, and everyone's mumbling about her," says Kevyn Aucoin, a New York makeup artist. "She feels like she should commit suicide."[3]

"We don't wake up for less than $10,000 a day," remarks Canadian-Italian supermodel Linda Evangelista pointedly.[4] She works 300 days a year, has more than 60 magazine covers to her credit between 1988 and 1991 alone, and is paid a minimum of $750 per hour for posing in fashion advertisements. Personal endorsements of fashion and cosmetic lines fetch her $500,000 each.[5] At least one major European fashion house reportedly paid Evangelista $20,000 for a single afternoon of modeling its clothes.[6]

"While the rest of the world has been slogging through a recession," remarks *Fortune* magazine, "an elite group of women including Naomi Campbell, Cindy Crawford, Linda Evangelista, Christy Turlington, and Claudia Schiffer have proved immune to the downturn."[7]

When asked by *Forbes* whether she was embarrassed at making a cool $2 million as a model last year, 23-year-old Christy Turlington replied, "There's a tremendous amount of money that's being made in this business [fashion and cosmetics], so when you think of it as being your commission, it's not that ridiculous."[8] As the "face" of Calvin Klein fragrances, she received about half a million dollars and pulled in another $1 million from other assorted modeling jobs, including doing runway work for Anne Klein and Perry Ellis—at $25,000 a day.[9] Sadly, as the twentieth century draws to a close, women can still earn more per hour by selling their bodies as models than they can by selling their skills.

With each passing season, the "look" changes. The latest trend is toward reed-like waifs—not va-va-voom models. Delicately beautiful and conspicuously curveless, the newest supermodels—such as Kate Moss, Kristen McMenemy, and Amber Valetta—are more reminiscent of bone-thin Twiggys than big-bosomed Barbie dolls.[10] These child-women, while praised by some top fashion experts, are criticized by others.

"It is weird that very tall, lanky women and anorexics can become symbols of beauty," remarks Donatella Girombelli, the head of an Italian fashion corporation.[11] Chris Athas, vice president of the National Association of Anorexia Nervosa and Associated Eating Disorders, finds the trend absolutely appalling. "It's a grotesque approach, this matter of hyping thinness in order to sell a different product," Athas says. "We're talking about emaciation again. Twiggy herself was anorexic and ill in her time."[12]

It isn't only adults who are influenced by today's high-fashion trends. All across the United States, there's also a burgeoning market for seductive, sultry designs aimed at toddlers and little girls: Baby Guess? Cutoff shorts and leopard-print midriff-baring blouses. Black chiffon skirts.

Gold lamé bikinis. When a slinky ensemble for young children, identical to one worn by Madonna on "Saturday Night Live," received rave reviews at a recent fashion show, buyers and parents instantly snapped them up. "People went nuts for those little Madonna outfits—they couldn't get enough of them," says Steven Cuba, designer for Artwear by Halley which manufactures clothes for girls under 10. "The woman who buys Escada and Chanel for herself flips when she sees something like it for her daughter."[13]

"Children's apparel designers used to be a year behind the [adult] industry," explained Rose Rosa of the Fashion Institute of Technology. "They can't do that anymore because kids and their parents have become so style conscious."[14]

Clothing and Empowerment

If there's any doubt that sex is on the minds of fashion editors, advertisers, designers, and merchandisers these days, consider: even *Ladies' Home Journal* has joined magazines like *New Woman* in emphasizing sex on its covers. That's because sex sells, according to Brad Mudge, a professor at the University of Colorado-Denver, as he explains why women's magazines contain so much of it. "They play up the role of female power as coming primarily through sex."[15] A recent article in an Atlanta newspaper announced that "young, leggy, sexy kittens are back," and offered the following examples as proof:

• television commericals for pants portray sexy women

saying "what they look for in a man's slacks";

•Calvin Klein ads featuring topless—and sometimes bottomless—women adorning the torsos of hunky men;

•Beer commercials featuring the blonde Swedish Bikini Team and statements such as "Why do men prefer blondes? <u>Dumb</u> question."

• a Bugle Boy jeans ad showing a man standing in his pants and stocking feet with a bare-legged woman dangling before him next to the caption, "Few things will make you want to take them off."[16]

"There are more ads that depict women as bimbos today than there were 15 years ago—after society has been revolutionized," asserts Linda Lazier-Smith, a professor at Ball State University in Indiana. She has examined advertising trends in *Ms., Time, Newsweek,* and *Playboy* since 1976.[17] Could it be because society has been revolutionized in other ways as well?

The result, says Ronald Collins, founder of the Center for the Study of Commercialism in Washington, D.C., is that Americans are schizophrenic, with one set of sexual standards in real life, and another in popular culture. "You go into the office, and the office is no, no, no. You're supposed to respect the dignity of women," Collins says. "But you go into the culture and it's yes, yes, yes. You're supposed to act on your basest instincts."[18]

Some women claim that clothing communicates their sexual power and boosts self-esteem, while also increasing their chances for success in today's highly competitive world. "The more empowered I am, the more I dress to please myself. There is no way one can divorce one's appearance from success," says Nadine Strossen, president of the American Civil Liberties Union. She also points out, "I guess some people might say I dress provocatively. But I've never had anyone treat me with disrespect. It has a lot to do with how you handle yourself."[19]

Yes, it does—and no, it doesn't. "There isn't a job in the world in which it's to your advantage to look bad, so do whatever is necessary to feel good about the way you present yourself," *Glamour* magazine recommended recently.[20] Sounds pretty good, really. But in a culture where sex sells and magazines convey the message that "female power . . . comes primarily through sex," looking *good* increasingly means looking *sexier.*

Commenting favorably on this trend in *Vogue,* Woody Hochswender offers a glimpse into what one is likely to encounter in the urban workplace today:

> She walked into the office. She wore sheer stockings on shaved legs, a blouse with enough buttons open to catch a cold. Her lips were red, her miniskirt black as sin.
>
> Sound like trouble? Or just a typical career look in the nineties?
>
> Why, the latter, of course. A dark slim skirt and a blouse open at the neck are wardrobe staples for working women in America today. The key missing piece, the woman's jacket—perhaps in a sharp color, with interesting buttons and a curvy, nipped-in waist—is probably hanging on a coat-rack somewhere waiting to go to lunch.
>
> Women at work have reclaimed their sexuality. Necklines are lower, colors are brighter, and skirts are shorter. Dresses are back and makeup is in. Many women executives say that fashion empowers them, makes them feel freer. Venus unchained. The new looks, they say, are a result of gaining credibility in the workplace and deciding

to use femininity to advantage. Why should a woman repress any aspect of her personality? Personal appeal—including a judicious use of sex appeal—is an unseen element in every social transaction. Use all your ammunition when you are at war, as one female executive put it. The brisk, sexless careerism of the 1980s is over.[21]

The gray-flannel-suit-and-floppy-silk-tie[22] boardroom concept of corporate fashion may be out—and that isn't all bad—but will seductive clothing ultimately help women achieve greater respect from male peers? Of course not. If anything, it's a significant step *backwards*. As a Christian and as a woman, I find this notion silly. What's so amazing is that the women who claim to be the most "liberated" are buying into it.

Clothing may not actually create boundary lines, but it definitely serves the purpose of reinforcing (or weakening) them. *Clothing choices have real-life consequences.* This can be easily illustrated. Given the choice, who would you prefer your mate working shoulder-to-shoulder with—a co-worker who employs her "femininity to advantage" through a "judicious use of sex appeal" in clothing, or one wearing an updated version of the gray flannel suit and a floppy silk foulard tie?

The Beautiful Princess

On the eve of July 29, 1981, I set my alarm for 4:00 A.M. Willing to forego an extra three hours of sleep, I wanted to watch Diana, daughter of the Earl of Spencer, marry Prince Charles. Beyond my desire to partake in this brief moment of British history, I wanted to see the princess' wedding dress. As it turned out, I wasn't disappointed.

Later, what especially impressed me about the Princess of Wales, besides her stunning smile, were her beautiful clothes. Rarely speaking on camera—I can recall hearing her voice only once, in a pre-wedding interview—the image of luxury conveyed by her attire and accessories spoke for her instead. Supposedly the most photographed person on earth during the eighties, Diana could spark a global reaction in the fashion world simply by wearing a new shade of blue, polka dots, or silk organza.

Before her marriage, Diana was noticeably pudgy, awkward, immature, and shy—"the insignificant ugly duckling [who] was obviously going to be a swan," according to her brother, Charles.[23] Her transformation from Knightsbridge nanny to royal sovereign was the essence of fairy tales. Her endless procession of dresses seemed to symbolize Diana's success in negotiating the difficult demands required of the monarchy. Accused of spending too much time and money on her wardrobe, Diana became the darling of the British fashion industry. If the empire was not impressed, young girls everywhere were. They oohed and aahed. While not a classic beauty, the princess nevertheless managed to become one of the most famous beauties in modern history. With one flash of her smile, the dream appeared real.

Until recently, most of the pictures of Princess Diana emphasized the glamour of her life, her evolving sense of style, and her wonderful warmth while performing charitable duties. Whether at a polo match or picking a child up from school, she looked absolutely wonderful from head to toe—especially in comparison to the rest of the Royal Family. (Her hats always look great.) Entire sections of books on Prince Charles and Princess Diana were devoted to her excellent taste in clothing. In retrospect, it now seems to mean something much different. Were the clothes a substitute for something else?

As reports of Diana's bulimia, depression, and desperate cries for help surfaced, I realized I should have known better than to believe a fairy tale. I found myself feeling sorry for the young woman who had been thrust onto a stage for which she was unprepared. Recently, while scanning a book about Diana's tenth wedding anniversary, I realized the clothes and her constant smile are what fooled me the most.

Blinded by Beauty

Images of women presented by fashion magazines, marketers, and princesses through clothing are an illusion. If we gaze upon these icons too long, the shadow is gradually substituted in our minds for reality. The fullness of our femininity—the cyclical rhythms of womanhood, the amount of body fat needed for healthy pregnancy and lactation, and the natural changes to our faces and figures over time—starts to feel strange, something to be fought off, rather than cherished and celebrated. Blinded by false images of beauty, we eventually end up failing to see our own.

Part 2 of this book discusses how we can recover our sight. But first, a few last thoughts on the subject of clothing—a subject near and dear to the hearts of many of us, considering the size of our wardrobes. In many ways, it would be much easier to renounce our closets once and for all and, like Mother Teresa, go about garbed in a white sari embellished with a few blue stripes. But for American women living in contemporary society, it wouldn't be culturally appropriate, and there's the rub.

I'm going to let you in on a little secret: apart from doing research or looking up a specific article, I avoid fashion magazines. I gave them up about five years ago and haven't regretted it since.

Growing up reading *Seventeen,* and later, *Glamour* and *Mademoiselle,* fashion magazines were a regular part of my life until I became a Christian. Removed from beauty culture's sphere of influence for a time while I was primarily at home with young children, I rarely wore makeup, and my wardrobe was basic.

Then, I started wearing cosmetics again, became an aerobics instructor, and began paying much more attention to what I ate and wore. I began reading fashion magazines occasionally. Slowly but surely, I started noticing the additional attention I received when I put extra effort and money into looking good. Sometimes it felt great. Even people at church often complimented me for improving my appearance. But sometimes it didn't feel great at all— it all seemed kind of empty. I rarely felt satisfied with myself or my wardrobe, became more tuned in to people noticing me, and was continually focused on controlling my weight.

I especially was aware of this I'm-not-good-enough feeling whenever I saw a particularly well-dressed woman, or looked at fashion magazines. Although I didn't subscribe to any, my husband's assistant at work started sending hers home with Dave for me to read after she was finished—all in all, worth about $30 each month. *What a deal,* I thought, *to be able to read all of these top publications for free.* The stack I received on a regular basis easily weighed 10 pounds.

Devouring each page, I told myself I was just reading for fun, but for several hours afterwards, I always felt tense and irritable. It took several months before I connected the magazines with the inner tension in my mind and spirit after I read them. (Some of us are pretty slow learners, I guess—especially when it comes to our own vanity.)

The more I thought about this, the more obvious it became. For me, reading women's fashion magazines is like my husband reading *Playboy* or *Penthouse*: it skews my perception of reality, makes me desire what isn't mine, and creates a gnawing dissatisfaction inside my heart about the things I do have—things the Lord has graciously provided for me.

After an evening of magazine-induced frustration, I realized that I, for one, can't read fashion magazines without "falling." This isn't spiritually neutral territory for me, but a destructive battle zone that has created real wounds. Consequently, I now avoid fashion magazines— not only out of obedience to the Holy Spirit's conviction, but out of a healthy fear and respect concerning what it does to my heart and head.

Recently, when a friend urged me to boycott a chain of convenience stores for selling *Playboy* and *Penthouse,* I asked her if she'd ever thought about boycotting magazines like *Vogue, Bazaar, Mirabella, Allure, Glamour, Seventeen, Mademoiselle,* and *Elle* as well. Their messages about women's sexuality are also spiritually harmful, I suggested to my friend, and equally potent in their ability to attack our birthright as believers—God's image in us.

While the message they carry may be more subtly attractive, it's every bit as soul-sickening. Make no mistake about this: the images they present are false.

As Christians, our clothing, cosmetics, hairstyles, and body sizes do not belong at the top of our personal agendas, but today's cult of beauty ruthlessly competes with Christ's lordship and continually seeks to place them there. Sure, we know these things are unimportant in light of eternity and aren't the true source of our beauty. But do we believe it in our hearts? If we measure our thoughts, tally the hours involved, and count the dollars we spend on clothes and beauty products and services, is the total amount significantly lower than the amount we're investing in God's Kingdom?

Scripture is clear: even the best clothing designs can't compete with the magnificent design of our bodies—yet often it's our clothing we feel the best about.[24] Jesus said, "Do not worry about your life, what you will eat or drink; or about your body, what you will wear. Is not life more important than food, and the body more important than clothes?" Then He asks, "Why do you worry about clothes?"[25] Why do we? Consider these questions:

• Most Christian women wear neither leather nor Lycra ® spandex, but clothing emphasizing body size and shape is common today, even at church. Is this something worth personally reevaluating?

• Is it appropriate for Christian women's groups to sponsor fashion shows, beauty seminars, and makeover workshops?

• What's the difference between *feminine* dressing and *sexual* dressing?

• Should Christians participate in beauty contests that compare women's clothes, makeup, and bodies even if talent and intelligence are scored by judges as well?

• If one side of the paying-attention-to-our-appearance pendulum is full participation in today's beauty culture, and the other is by wearing no makeup or external "adornment" at all, are there spiritual traps involved in *both* of these extremes?

By identifying ways that social ideals and expectations influence us, and then putting beauty in its proper place in our lives, small seeds of truth are planted and our ability to fully function in the Lord's strength, freedom, and grace grows. We've been stunted by beauty's lies long enough. Now that we've diagnosed the problem, are we ready for the cure?

Action Plan

Building a Professional Wardrobe

Business image consultant Susan Bixler of Atlanta suggests the following $500 wardrobe starter-kit to women on a budget, who are going to work outside the home or after graduating from college:

• black suit ($140);

• taupe or olive suit ($100);

• cobalt blue suit ($95);

- red jacket ($75);

- blouse, quality polyester or silk ($40);

- black leather pumps ($30);

- panty hose, five pairs ($10);

- faux pearl or gold earrings ($10).[26]

Use your personal preferences to guide you in selecting a basic "kit" of interchangeable work wear, based on Bixler's guide.

For a classic look, a well-tailored jacket with knee-length skirt, a simple blouse or fine-gauge knit sweater, an understated necklace and earrings, leather handbag, and pumps, work well together. A tailored wardrobe doesn't have to cost a fortune. You can shop the sales, consignment stores, and outlet or discount stores.

You really can find the basics at an affordable price. Last year, I bought $1,096 worth of name-brand black-and-white jackets, blouses, slacks, and skirts for $187 at Macy's spring sale. I got a much-needed wardrobe change at a fraction of the original price.

Jackets, suits, and coordinated separates are very practical and appropriate, even if you don't work outside the home. In addition to writing and speaking-related events, I've worn these outfits to school board meetings, legislative hearings, formal church functions, and dinners with my husband's co-workers. Some might argue suits and coordinates may not be as feminine as fancy dresses, but given our culture, I think it's wise to dress in a no-nonsense yet pleasant-looking way when we're trying to do or say something valuable.

Evaluating Your Wardrobe

As an interesting exercise, go through your closet and assess the fitness of each garment for your lifestyle.

• List everything that's in your closet and dresser. Record what you spent on the clothes, jewelry, and accessories that are in season and add up the items in your inventory. Repeat this step for each season, adding and subtracting from the list as necessary.

If you've already made a significant investment in this area, there may be little need to continue investing much money in your wardrobe except for occasional purchases to replace worn or outdated items. If you find that you haven't invested enough, plan your budget to allow you to purchase a few key items within the next few months.

• Think about the image you want to project through the clothing and accessories you own. Is there anything that you'd like to change? If so, make a plan for getting rid of things that you no longer will wear; decide when and with what you can replace these items.

• Do your clothes enhance or detract from your Christian witness? Knowing that clothing communicates, write down what you would like to "say" to others about yourself—and your relationship to the Lord—through your clothing choices. When you shop, take the list with you and carefully consider your choices.

Eventually, you'll find that regularly evaluating your wardrobe according to these steps will produce excellent results. This plan has freed me from preoccupation with what I wear and has enabled me to forget about my clothes, once they're on, so that I can think about other things. (I'm also spending far less money and shopping less frequently, a fact my husband and I *both* appreciate.)

It's not a rigid system, but one that creates pleasant, reasonable boundary lines for how many clothes to buy and how much to pay.

❧ *Focus Questions* ❧

1. To what degree should a biblical understanding of visual lust influence clothing choice? In what ways can that understanding help us dress in ways that play down the body rather than displaying it?

2. Do you think you've gone too far in adopting contemporary clothing fashions? If so, what would you change?

3. What is modesty? How is its message communicated by our behavior as well as by the beauty ideals we emulate?

Part Two

The Cure

❧ Seven ❧

Beauty and the Bible

A mere notice of the influence of personal beauty alone, on individuals and on society, in all ages of the world, would embrace the whole history of the human race. It has, perhaps, owing to the lawless passions and vices of mankind, been productive of more contention than has been caused by ambition, and more misery than has been occasioned by avarice and gold.
—— *A. J. Colley,* The Toilet and Cosmetic Arts in Ancient and Modern Times, *1866*

It is amazing how complete is the delusion that beauty is goodness.
—— *Leo Tolstoy,* The Kreutzer Sonata, *1889*

If someone asked you what the Bible says about beauty, what would you say?

I don't know about you, but what I grew up *thinking* the Bible says about beauty, compared to what it *really* says, never quite matched. Raised in a Christian home, I was nonetheless taught by my family and friends that appearance was of paramount importance. While growing up, the clothes I wore, the accessories I picked, and the way my hair looked were all expected to be just so. Even when I rebelled and began wearing miniskirts and Twiggy-type makeup, I was still living out the values I had acquired earlier.

I don't know where or when this emphasis on beauty began. I know it wasn't with my grandmother. She was a woman who spent little time on her appearance. In Grandma's time, women rarely finished high school, worked hard, married young, didn't drive, and wouldn't think of traveling alone—you know, way back when the divorce rate was only about five percent instead of 50. I don't remember Grandma wearing much makeup, if any, and her clothes were typically plain for women of that era. Her beauty advice mostly consisted of telling me to sit up straight and not to eat too many potatoes.

As if to defy all of this dreary domestic dullness, as a

teenager my mother took up the cause of beauty with a vengeance. She began modeling clothes at a local dress shop and rarely missed a beat thereafter. Mom's style and sensibilities about fashion were acted out daily, as a way of life, rather than occasional flights of fancy. While wonderfully tasteful most of the time, she subtly conveyed the message to both my sisters and me that *how* you look is an important part of *who* you are.

It wasn't only my mother who convinced me that appearance counts. Most of the older women I knew worried about the way they looked. My godmother, Janie, went to the beauty parlor regularly to have her blonde hair bleached; neighbors on all sides talked about who weighed what and how people looked; and ladies at church constantly compared themselves to one another. Thinking back on my childhood, I can remember only one woman who did otherwise—my Girl Scout leader, Mrs. Swart. From her I learned that hiking, helping others, building campfires, and singing folk songs could be more fun than spending all my time curling my hair or fixing my face.

These days, in an age of looks-obsession that's so all-encompassing you can't even grab a gallon of milk at the grocery store without being peppered by multiple images of sexy supermodels and a slew of beauty-speak, things haven't gotten any better. From what I can tell, only nuns, radical feminists, and isolated members of conservative religious sects choose to completely ignore the dictates of today's beauty culture.

What began as a trickle of beauty ideals and expectations in the '20s and '30s became a veritable torrent in the '60s and '70s. It sweeps over us today like a gigantic tidal wave. Contemporary beauty culture reaches out to touch every one of us. Few can resist its grip entirely.

To reject this mindset can be costly: why would any woman want to look plain (i.e., bad) when looking pretty (i.e., good) is now such a major part of what life is all about?[1]

As Grandma's generation passes away, the generations following display an ever-increasing preoccupation with beauty. Kids these days take it for granted that they need to look a certain way, wear the right clothes, and have their hair permed—all before they're eight years old. These days we rarely meet a young girl or teenager (or preschooler!) who isn't concerned about these things. My daughters belong to the third generation of American women to place a high value on appearance. When at age 14 they began using hairspray to spritz bangs even Woody Woodpecker would envy, I couldn't help wondering: *Where did I go wrong?*

Somehow, somewhere, between our grandmothers' generation and our own, we exchanged simplicity for sophistication. For most of us, it's only the size of our wallets that keeps us from investing even more money in looking better.

What the Bible Says

The Bible—not our culture, families, peer groups, or church traditions—gives us the truth we need to see beyond these falsehoods to reality. Only Jesus can set us free from worrying about the way we look, making us who He would have us be through the work of the Holy

Spirit. God's love—not our husbands', fathers', mothers', sisters', brothers', or friends'—enables us to accept ourselves the way He's made us and to appreciate the goodness of His image made real in us for eternity: "being confident of this, that he who began a good work in you will carry it on to completion until the day of Jesus Christ."[2]

Before writing this book, I'd rarely thought about beauty as a biblical subject. But it's definitely there—a complex theme balanced by enough ambiguity to keep us all thinking for quite some time. How many of us, for example, have ever noticed that the first biblical passage referring to beauty ends in a curse? That the Creation story never describes Eve's appearance? Or the fact that beauty in the Bible is consistently connected to trouble and temptation far more often than it is to blessing and goodness?

Though I'm far from being a bona fide Bible scholar, I think you'll find the following discussion to be an interesting starting point for your own in-depth study. On the one hand, it's clear the Bible dismisses physical beauty as fleeting, an aspect of the human body destined to perish "as the flower of the grass."[3] On the other hand, Song of Songs unabashedly declares the ecstasy of finding one's beloved attractive—"How beautiful you are, my darling! Oh, how beautiful!"—in its rapturous celebration of married love. While beauty is evident everywhere in God's glorious creation,[4] the Bible also warns against beauty as a snare.[5]

Perhaps part of the reason for this paradox is because physical beauty and spiritual beauty are not the same thing, though in many people's minds they are linked together—a concept acquired from the teachings of Greek and Roman mythology, romantic poets, and fairy tales.

Let's put the record straight. No matter what we believe about what the Bible says about physical beauty, it never instructs women (or men, for that matter) to desire it, nor does it necessarily depict beauty as a blessing for those who have it.

As with other unique qualities God gives to people, beauty is shown in the Bible to be a physical attribute God occasionally uses to further His purposes—as in the case of Esther, for example—but beauty is definitely not something the Bible instructs us to wish for, ask for, strive for, or believe in. That's an idea our culture has picked up from other sources. Put simply, the notion that looking beautiful equates with being beautiful (or that being beautiful makes one look beautiful), is false from a biblical point of view.

In Scripture, physical beauty is never used as a metaphor for goodness or counted as any kind of moral virtue. In spite of the fairy tales, beauty has no magical power of its own to make bad people good. The beautiful princess who kisses the frog cannot turn him into a prince no matter how hard she tries.

What Disney's versions of *Sleeping Beauty, Cinderella, The Little Mermaid, Snow White,* and *Beauty and the Beast* are selling successfully to children today are just updated expressions of a very old myth—a belief that's deeply rooted in pagan folklore rather than in Christian teaching and tradition.

The myth is this: because beauty is good, it can conquer evil. In many fairy tales, beauty is portrayed as possessing spiritual power—a kind of power that comes from a source other than knowing, serving, and surrendering to the lordship of Jesus Christ. In fact, the original meaning of the word *glamour* described a type of enchantment used by witches—such as the one used by Morgana in the tales of King Arthur—when they wanted to appear to be someone else. Other words used in reference to women's beauty clearly demonstrate a connection to magic as well, including the words *alluring, captivating, charming, enchanting, entrancing, beguiling, bewitching,* and *fascinating.*

The mythical power of beauty reminds me more of an early scene in *The Wizard of Oz* than anything the Bible teaches. When the dazzling Glenda asks Dorothy, "Are you a good witch or a bad witch?" isn't she really telling us about two different types of sorceresses—the good witches, who are bright, beautiful, and cast nice spells, and the bad witches, who are dark, ugly, and cast terrible spells? Popular fairy tale heroines do not oppose the dark side with the power of God. What they use could be called white magic or sorcery.

Make no mistake: from the standpoint of Scripture, it doesn't matter what a sorceress "looks" like. If a story shows beauty changing people, we should simply ask, "How?" Most fairy tales depict a "good witch" solution, not Christian salvation, as the cure for curses. Yet, according to the Bible, it took the horror of our Lord's crucifixion to turn bad people into good ones—not a blessed beauty's benevolence. As Christians, we know from Scripture that Jesus alone is truly good. Spiritual power is not ours to wield as we wish.

Beauty's Daughters

As the influence of today's beauty culture grows stronger and becomes increasingly more powerful around the world, it's important to understand what this myth really represents. First articulated by Plato, it suggests that goodness and physical beauty are identical.[6]

As sociologist Anthony Synnott explains:

> The beauty mystique, in its simplest form, is the belief that the beautiful is good, and the ugly is evil; and conversely, that the morally good is physically beautiful (or "good-looking") and the evil is ugly. Thus the physical and the metaphysical, body and soul, appearance and reality, inner and outer are one. Each mirrors the other. The belief is most ancient.[7]

God's Word proves this belief to be false. Over and over again, physical beauty is shown in Scripture to be a skin-deep quality distinctly separate from the condition of one's heart.

In its first reference to physical beauty, the Bible offers a dramatic illustration of this truth:

> When men began to increase in number on the earth and daughters were born to them, the sons of God saw that the daughters of men were beautiful, and they married any of them they chose. Then the Lord said, "My Spirit will not contend with man forever, for he is mortal; his days will be a hundred and twenty years."
>
> The Nephilim were on the earth in those days—and also afterward—when the sons of God went to the daughters of men and had children by them. They were the heroes of old, men of renown.
>
> The Lord saw how great man's wickedness had become, and that every inclination of the thoughts of his heart was only evil all the time. The Lord was grieved that he had

made man on the earth and his heart was filled with pain. So the Lord said, "I will wipe mankind, whom I have created, from the face of the earth—men and animals, and creatures that move along the ground, and birds of the air—for I am grieved that I have made them." But Noah found favor in the eyes of the Lord.[8]

Though the actual identity of the "sons of God" and "daughters of men" continues to be debated, one thing in this passage is plain: God-created physical beauty, and spiritual or moral goodness, are not one and the same. On the contrary. Given the intense reaction men normally have toward it, the presence of physical beauty can make it more difficult for goodness to predominate in a woman's life, not less![9]

The beauty of the daughters mentioned in Genesis appears to have played a direct role in causing these men and women to commit unlawful acts of intercourse, with dire consequences for everyone: the destruction of mankind by the Flood. Here, beauty is clearly linked with sin, not goodness. Thousands of years later, the intimate connection between beauty, temptation, and lust is still going strong.

Thorns in the Desert

The subject of beauty comes up in the Old Testament again after Abraham (called Abram in this passage) and his wife, Sarah (here called Sarai), have left home and are heading through the desert toward Canaan. Re-routed in transit due to famine in the land, Abraham seems to suddenly realize that entering Egypt could present serious problems for the two of them traveling together:

> As he was about to enter Egypt, he said to his wife Sarai, "I know what a beautiful woman you are. When the Egyptians see you, they will say, 'This is his wife.' Then they will kill me but will let you live. Say you are my sister, so that I will be treated well for your sake and my life will be spared because of you." [10]

Sarah's beauty was evidently so striking that upon arriving in Egypt, she quickly came to the notice of the Pharaoh's officials and was taken to live with him at the palace. Treated with favor as Sarah's "brother" (he was in fact her half-brother as well as her husband), Abraham grew phenomenally rich, but when the Lord inflicted serious diseases on Pharaoh and his household as a result of the deception, the truth of their marital relationship finally became known.

"What have you done to me?" we can almost hear Pharaoh crying after discovering how he'd been tricked. "Why didn't you tell me she was your wife? Why did you say, 'She is my sister,' so that I took her to be my wife? Now then, here is your wife. Take her and go!" [11]

In this story, beauty is once again directly associated with sin. Lying, greed, fear of murder, adultery, and exile are all parts of the picture Sarah's beauty paints. And, as if this weren't enough, almost the entire scenario gets repeated again. The next time around, it's King Abimelech who takes Sarah into his court, but the Lord appears to him in a dream and adultery is providentially avoided. [12] Throughout Sarah's stay in the king's household, however, none of the women are able to bear children. It isn't until Abraham confesses and prays to God for help that Abimelech's household is healed.

What a mess! Because of Sarah's beauty, Abraham believes he'll be killed: unable to trust God to deliver him, he uses deceit and deception (make that two deceptions) to avoid this dreadful scenario. We're never told that God gave this idea to Abraham. It's impossible, in fact, for the Lord to instruct someone to sin; rather, the extent of God's mercy and faithfulness to His covenant with Abraham is revealed instead. At all times, the situation is described as a plan of Abraham's own making, followed by an unhappy chain of consequences for both of the affected households—including an encore performance by Abraham's son, Isaac.[13]

These three similar stories underscore the ability of beauty to provoke pain even as we marvel at its power: how could any woman be so beautiful that a king might be willing to kill for her?

Later on, we're shown exactly how. One evening, while King David is walking on the roof of his palace in Jerusalem, he looks down and spies upon his neighbor's residence. Seeing an extraordinarily beautiful woman named Bathsheba taking her monthly *mikvah*—a menstrual purification bath—he quickly sends a messenger to bring her to the palace for his pleasure:

> From the roof he saw a woman bathing. The woman was very beautiful and David sent someone to find out about her. The man said, "Isn't this Bathsheba, the daughter of Eliam and the wife of Uriah the Hittite?" Then David sent messengers to get her. She came to him, and he slept with her.[14]

After going to bed together, Bathsheba became pregnant and David placed her husband, Uriah, on the front line of battle where he could be quickly killed. Later,

Uriah's untimely death is followed by yet another: the loss of the baby boy born to Bathsheba and David.[15]

In the course of this story, we witness the breaking of not one or two, but almost all of the 10 Commandments as David covets his neighbor's wife, steals Bathsheba away from her home, commits adultery, plots against his neighbors, plans Uriah's murder, dishonors the teaching of his parents, and exalts his own position of authority above God's—a tragedy of great proportions which affects not only David's immediate family, but the future course of Israel as well.

Other accounts of beautiful women in the Bible also teach that physical attractiveness isn't to be considered "good" in and of itself. Rebekah, for example, conspired against her husband to acquire the birthright for her second-born son, Jacob.[16] In the course of time, her beautiful daughter-in-law, Rachel, stole statues of false gods from her father and then lied to Jacob about having them.[17]

"Happily ever after" isn't beauty's end in these tales. On the contrary, we find lying, cheating, stealing, murder, conniving, adultery, and idol worship linked to beauty instead—all in all, a very human (and not very pretty) list of actions unredeemed by beauty's presence.

Esther

The one shining example of God's use of beauty to fulfill His purposes can be found in the story of Esther. A young Jewish girl raised by her uncle Mordecai after her parents' death, she is "discovered" in a kingdom-wide beauty contest. Before being taken to the palace, Mordecai instructs Esther not to reveal her nationality. Later, he keeps in touch with his niece by frequently strolling near the harem's courtyard and asking how she's doing.

Prior to being presented to King Xerxes, Esther is required to complete a full year of beauty treatments: six months with oil of myrrh, and six with perfumes and cosmetics. When they meet, the king is more attracted to Esther than to any of the other women in his harem, and he makes her his queen. But this is the sugary stuff of romance novels, *not* biblical heroes. As the plot thickens, it becomes evident that Queen Esther is there for a better reason than to be royally pampered as one of the king's pets.

When the king's highest official, Haman, sends out a decree in Xerxes' name in a murderous plot to annihilate the Jews, Mordecai rips his clothes and goes about the city in sackcloth and ashes, "wailing loudly and bitterly."[18] Unable to enter the king's gate in such a state, Mordecai sends a copy of Haman's phony edict to Esther and urges her to beg the king for mercy. When she responds that she could be put to death for approaching the king in his inner court without being summoned, the unwaveringly devout uncle responds:

> Do not think that because you are in the king's house you alone of all the Jews will escape. For if you remain silent at this time, relief and deliverance for the Jews will arise from another place, but you and your father's family will perish. And who knows but that you have come to royal position for such a time as this?[19]

After much prayer and fasting, Esther wisely intervenes at exactly the right moment, resulting in Haman's execution. Then, Xerxes gives Esther Haman's entire estate and issues a new edict granting Jews throughout his kingdom the right to assemble and protect themselves in exchange for Haman's decree of death. Today the Jewish celebration of Purim is an annual observance of God's sovereign deliverance for the Hebrew nation. Marked by "days of feasting and joy and giving presents of food to one another and gifts to the poor," it was first instituted by Esther's uncle Mordecai nearly 2,500 years ago.[20]

It was Esther's obedience to God and the Lord's sovereign intervention—not Esther's beauty—that brought about Haman's timely defeat. Even Mordecai was assured of this: if Esther hadn't cooperated, he believed God had planned another way to deliver his people. But Esther made the right choice. By placing her trust in God, she was given the necessary wisdom to accomplish the greater good of her nation.

Esther's legendary looks didn't have spiritual power to transform evil in her husband or her country, though that's what countless fairy tales teach. Esther's beauty, as powerful as it was, served a much different purpose: it brought the king's attention to a woman who loved and obeyed God. In all of the times feminine beauty is referred to in the Bible, only two women described as being beautiful—Esther and Abigail—are consistently pictured as serving the Lord and doing good.

Different Types of Beauty

Although modern English versions of the Bible commonly use the word *beauty* to refer to several kinds of beauty, Hebrew and Greek words make a clearer distinction between them. Looking at these words enriches our ability to talk about and understand their different meanings. For example, the most frequently used word to describe beautiful women in the Bible, *yapheh*, is different from the Hebrew word reserved for "the most beautiful of all," *towb*:

> **beautiful:** *yapheh* (yaw-feh'). This is the word used to describe Sarah, Rachel, David, Abigail, Absalom, Absalom's sister Tamar, Absalom's daughter Tamar, Abishag, and Job's daughters. (See Genesis 12:11; Genesis 29:17; 1 Samuel 14:27; 1 Samuel 16:12; 1 Samuel 25:3; 2 Samuel 13:1; 2 Samuel 14:25; 1 Kings 1:4; and Job 42:15, respectively.) The primary root for *yapheh* literally means to be bright. Interestingly, *yapheh* is used in the Bible to describe the beauty of both men and women.

> **good:** *towb* (tobe). It means to be beautiful in the widest sense—beautiful, best, better, bountiful, fair, glad, gracious, loving, pleasant, pleasing, sweet, and well-favored. In English, the closest equivalent to *towb* might be *gorgeous*, which means splendid or sumptuous in appearance, coloring, etc., or extremely enjoyable.[21] *Towb* is the word used to describe the beauty of the "daughters of men," Rebekah, Bathsheba, and Esther. (Genesis 6:2; Genesis 24:16; 2 Samuel 11:2 and Esther 2:7.) Given the previous stories concerning these biblical beauties, however, it should be noted that *towb* doesn't mean that a person is also spiritually or morally good.

Additional words used to describe physical beauty in the Bible, and specific examples, include:

> **beauty:** *yophiy* (yof-ee'). Charm is deceptive and *beauty* is fleeting; but a woman who fears the Lord is to be praised (Proverbs 31:30).

> **shapely:** *mareh* (mar-eh'). Leah had weak eyes, but Rachel

was *lovely in form,* and beautiful (Genesis 29:17).

beautiful figure or form: *toar* (to'-ar). This girl, who was also known as Esther, was *lovely in form* and features . . . (Esther 2:7).

very beautiful: *yepheh-phiyah* (yef-eh' fee-yaw'). Egypt is a *beautiful* heifer, but a gadfly is coming against her from the north (Jeremiah 46:20).

lovely, becoming: *naveh* (naw-veh'). Dark am I, yet *lovely,* O daughters of Jerusalem . . . (Song of Songs 1:5).

comely, pleasant, beautiful: *naah* (naw-aw'). Your cheeks are *beautiful* with earrings, your neck with strings of jewels (Song of Songs 1:10).

pleasing, agreeable, delightful: *noam* (no'-am). How beautiful you are and how *pleasing,* O love, with your delights! (Song of Songs 7:6).

vision, appearance: *mareh* (mar-eh'). He had no *beauty* or majesty to attract us to him, nothing in his appearance that we should desire him (Isaiah 53:2).

In a distinctly separate category, the word for beauty used in English Bibles sometimes refers to *ornamental beauty* or *adornment* [22]—the signs and accessories of beauty rather than physical beauty itself. Whether it's obtained by wearing a jewel-encrusted bracelet or gold-toned eyeshadow, this is the kind of beauty women "put on"—the aspect of appearance acquired through the accoutrements of cosmetics, jewelry, hairstyle, and clothing. It's this type of beauty Peter used to describe elements of women's appearance in his first epistle.

ornamental beauty: *tiphereth* (tif-eh'reth). Beauty, splendor, bravery, honor, fair, comely, glorious, and majestic are all aspects of this word, which also refers to adorned beauty. (See, for example, 2 Chronicles 3:6; Psalm 96:6; Isaiah 28:5;

Isaiah 64:11; Lamentations 2:1; Ezekiel 23:42.)

beauty, adornment, attractiveness: *kosmeo* (kos-meh'-o). The Greek word, *kosmeo,* from where we get the English word *cosmetics,* means to put in proper order; to decorate, garnish, adorn, or trim. It's also related to the words *kosmikos* (kos-mee-kos'), which translates into English as *cosmic* or *worldly,* and *kosmos* (kos'-mos), which means an orderly arrangement, cosmos, or the world. *Kosmeo* is the word often translated into English as beauty in 1 Peter 3:3-5, but in the King James Version, it's translated as *adornment* or *adorn,* which means to decorate or add beauty to, or to make pleasing, more attractive, or more impressive.

In contrast to *physical* beauty and *adorned* beauty, the Bible shows us a *beauty of holiness* which belongs to the Lord:

beauty of holiness: *hadar* (haw-dawr') or *hadarah* (had-aw-raw'). Translated into English as magnificence, honor, majesty, beauty, comeliness, excellency, glory, or goodly, the primary root of this word means to swell up (i.e., magnify), implying favor or honor. (See its use in 1 Chronicles 16:29; 2 Chronicles 20:21; Job 40:10; Psalm 29:2; Psalm 96:9; and Psalm 110:3.) For example: One thing I ask of the Lord, this is what I seek: that I may dwell in the house of the Lord all the days of my life, to gaze upon the *beauty* of the Lord and to seek him in his temple (Psalm 27:4, italics added).

Other words used in the Bible to demonstrate the beauty of God's holiness are *radiance, glory, resplendent, shine,* and *splendor.* It's rare for anyone to encounter this type of supernatural splendor here on earth. But one day, when we see Jesus face to face, we'll see for ourselves the beauty of His holiness.

Even still, we're given a small foretaste of this delightful pleasure today. When the Apostle Paul wrote that "we, who with unveiled faces all reflect the Lord's glory, are being transformed into his likeness with ever-increasing glory, which comes from the Lord, who is the Spirit,"[23] I think this is the kind of beauty that he was talking about. Every Christian carries this spark of God's great beauty, no matter what they may "look" like.

Beauty Beyond Belief

After completing a biblical word study on beauty, one striking fact stands out: the majority of the women in Scripture aren't described as beautiful.

We aren't told, for example, what Ruth looked like, though many of us picture her as being pretty, or how Jesus' mother, Mary, appeared. In fact, in the New Testament, there's no reference to women's physical attractiveness at all! Pretty remarkable, isn't it? Yet how often do we picture Mary of Bethany, Priscilla, Joanna, or even Elizabeth as being unattractive looking? If you are having a hard time believing me, check these references for yourself.

Anna: Luke 2:36-37

Apphia: Philemon 2

Chloe: 1 Corinthians 1:11

Damaris: Acts 17:34

Dorcas/Tabitha: Acts 9:36-42

Elizabeth: Luke 1:5-22, 39-45, 56-58

Eunice: 2 Timothy 1:4

Jairus' daughter: Matthew 9:18-25; Mark 5:21-43; Luke 8:40-56

Joanna: Luke 8:3, 24:1-11

Julia: Romans 16:15

Junias: Romans 16:7

Lois: 2 Timothy 1:4

Lydia: Acts 16:14-15, 40

Martha: Luke 10:38-41; John 11:1-27; John 12:2

Mary Magdalene: Matthew 27:55-61, 28:1-11; Mark 15:40-41, 47, 16:1-11; Luke 8:2, 10:38-41, 23:55-24:10; John 19:25, 20:1-18

Mary of Bethany: John 11:1-45; John 12:1-7

Mary, a Christian worker: Romans 16:6

Mary, Jesus' Mother: Matthew 1:18-24, 2:11; Luke 1:27-56, 2:1-7, 16-52; John 19:25-27; Acts 1:14.

Mary, the mother of James: Matthew 27:55-61; Mark 15:40-16:8; Luke 24:10

Mary, the wife of Clopas: John 19:25

Nereus' sister: Romans 16:15

Olympas: Romans 16:15

Persis: Romans 16:12

Peter's mother-in-law: Matthew 8:14-15; Mark 1:29-31; Luke 4:38-39

Philip's daughters: Acts 21:9

Phoebe: Romans 16:1

Priscilla: Acts 18:2-3,18-26; Romans 16:3; 1 Corinthians 16:19; Timothy 4:19

Rufus' mother: Romans 16:13

Samaritan woman: John 4:1-26, 39

Salome: Mark 15:40-41, 16:1-8

Susanna: Luke 8:3

Syrophenician (Canaanite) woman: Matthew 15:21-28; Mark 7:24-30

Tryphena: Romans 16:15

Tryphosa: Romans 16:15

Widow of Nain: Luke 7:12-15

Woman described by Luke as a "sinner": Luke 7:36-50

Woman taken in adultery: John 7:53-8:11

Woman with a hemorrhage: Matthew 9:20-22; Mark 5:25-34; Luke 8:43-48

The omission of beauty as a measure of a woman's worth in the New Testament stands in striking contrast to the Old, given the number of times women's appearances are cited in each section. I don't believe this is merely an oversight. *By never bringing up what women looked like, but telling us about their inner qualities, personal relationships, and love for the Lord instead, the New Testament provides us with a uniquely Christian perspective upon which to build our identity as women*—one that doesn't measure our worth by the beauty of our faces, the shape of our bodies, the style of our hair, the brand of our cosmetics, the fit of our clothing, or the way we attract others.

If we believe what the Bible says about this subject, physical beauty is a non-issue for believers—so why do we pay homage to it? How many people who claim that "it's what's inside that counts" truly believe it? Here, in the New Testament's only discourse on beauty, we're reminded of that statement's truth:

> *Your beauty should not come from outward adornment,* such as braided hair and the wearing of gold jewelry and fine clothes. *Instead, it should be that of your inner self,* the unfading beauty of a gentle and quiet spirit,*which is of great worth in God's sight.* [24]

This is it! A kind of beauty that lasts forever, one that won't fade "as the flowers of the grass" with the passing of seasons, but grows ever brighter with the passage of time—a reflection of Christ's own lordship within us. A kind of beauty hidden inside our hearts, fashioned within us supernaturally by God. A kind of beauty that can't be physically put on, made up, covered over, or taken off, but is 100 percent *real*. A kind of beauty the Bible declares "of great worth in God's sight"—contained not in our faces and bodies, but created deep within us at "the inmost center of our beings" by our Maker.

What would happen if we took this truth seriously? If we gave up our worries and anxieties and fears about the way we look—and based our ideals and expectations on God's opinion about beauty instead of on our culture's?

It's a fact: no matter how hard we try, we can never make ourselves beautiful where it counts the most. Only Jesus can. Often the things we use to beautify ourselves distract our attention from what Christ's beauty is all about: the fruit of His Spirit brought to bear in our spirits, reaching the world for the glory of God's Kingdom, changing every aspect of our hearts and minds and lives.

Action Plan

A Biblical View of Beauty

On the days when you're tempted to return to your old ways of seeing and doing things related to beauty, try reading a few of the following passages of Scripture— and any other applicable verses you find along the way— to get back on track. You may also want to copy several down in a journal and write out your responses.

- Psalms 19:7-14, 23:1-3; 25:1-15; 34:1-9; 86; 121; 139; 145:8-21
- Proverbs 3:5-8; 31:30
- Isaiah 40:28-31; 43:1-2; 57:15-19; 61:1-3, 10
- Matthew 6:25-34; 11:28-29
- John 15:1-17
- Romans 8:1-4
- 2 Corinthians 3:17-4:7
- Ephesians 2:4-10
- Philippians 2:1-16
- Colossians 2:6-8
- Hebrews 12:2-3
- James 4:7-10
- 1 Peter 1:3-9; 5:6-11

Protect Your Mind

If you feel self-pity or condemnation about your appearance after watching the latest diet drink commercial, or if you get depressed while shopping for a new bathing suit, pray for protection of your mind and heart and recall the truth about who you are and what the Lord is doing in the "inmost center of your being." Remember, the King has called you by name. Praise Him for the beauty He alone can give—the only kind that lasts forever!

❧ *Focus Questions* ❧

1. Before reading this chapter, how would you have described what the Bible says about beauty? Is your perspective any different now? What surprised you most in studying this topic?

2. In what ways were beauty ideals and expectations passed down to you in your family? Was your appearance emphasized frequently? If so, how were you affected? If not, did you ever feel left out or criticized by people outside your family as a result? What impact did it have on you?

3. Why does the belief that physical beauty is desirable and equals *good* continue to permeate our society?

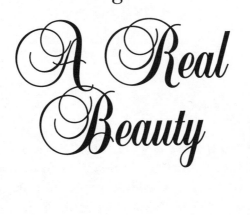

Eight

A Real Beauty

*It is a serious thing to live in a society of possible gods
and goddesses, to remember that the dullest and most
uninteresting person you talk to may one day be a creature which, if you saw it now, you would be strongly
tempted to worship, or else a horror and a corruption
such as you now meet, if at all, only in a nightmare. All
day long, we are, in some degree, helping each other to
one of these destinations. It is in the light of these overwhelming possibilities, it is with the awe and circumspec-
tion proper to them, that we should conduct all our deal-
ings with one another, all friendships, all loves, all play,
all politics. There are no ordinary people. You have never
talked to a mere mortal.*

—— *C. S. Lewis, 1898-1963*

*Her walk was ever close with God, whose light was in the
holy beauty of her face.*

—— *From the epitaph of Emma Allen Bates
(December 17, 1842—January 13, 1923), Oakland Cemetery,
Atlanta, Georgia.*

$\mathcal{W}$ho are the most beautiful women in the world? *Harper's Bazaar* ranked America's top 10 beauties as Demi Moore, Anjelica Huston, Robin Wright, Laura Dern, Geena Davis, Naomi Campbell, Debra Winger, Paulina Porizkova, Vanessa Williams, and Iman. *People Weekly's* recent list of the 50 most beautiful people includes Michelle Pfeiffer, Cindy Crawford, Whitney Houston, Kate Moss, Janine Turner, and Bridget Fonda. The Miss World USA pageant picked its top three candidates last week; Miss America will soon follow with its selection in September. Next year, and the year after that, and the years after that, a new wave of beauties will sweep these faces to the sidelines, offering the latest contestants the title of superstar in a world where what's "in fashion" changes regularly.

Beautiful women turn up everywhere these days. This weekend, while strolling through a local mall, the Atlanta Hawks cheerleading squad was on hand to autograph team posters and enthusiastically greet Dave and me outside J. C. Penney. At church yesterday morning, I saw a stunning-looking woman who appeared to be wearing apparel, accessories, and jewelry worth at least $25,000 glide gracefully into a pew in front of me, temporarily interrupting the hymn-singing of several surrounding parishioners. Earlier today, while taking my niece to her departure gate at Hartsfield International Airport, a gorgeous young blonde woman in a midriff-baring nylon aerobics outfit nonchalantly stood next to Kristin and me on the underground transit as men nearby tried not to act stupid.

Tonight, I think I'll find a good book, pour myself an ice-cold glass of lemonade, and hide my television in the closet.

Uncommonly Beautiful

Defining real beauty has never been easy. Some say real beauty consists of the way a woman looks; others claim it's how she acts. Most people say its both. Still others, myself included, argue that the best kind of beauty—the type that lasts *forever*—often appears to be something else entirely: it usually comes to us in disguise, and rarely reaches full bloom before the age of 65.

To be sure, there's an exquisite type of natural physical beauty 99 percent of the world's population will never attain—a fleeting physical beauty many call "perfect." Characterized by a pleasing symmetry of face and form, youthful appearance, sexual attractiveness, healthy vitality, and a near-universal acceptance of its existence, it represents the centuries-old pinnacle of the beauty hierarchy.

Liz Taylor and Grace Kelley had this type of beauty; Marilyn Monroe didn't. We see its portrayal in Botticelli's painting of *Venus*, yet it eludes us in the enigmatic smile of daVinci's *Mona Lisa*. In the sixties, Jean Shrimpton demonstrated she had it, whereas Twiggy only pretended to. This year, only a handful of baby girls around the world will gain entry at birth into this elite echelon—and will consequently struggle with the adulation and envy of almost everyone they meet for the rest of their lives.

Hundreds of years from now, photos of Liz Taylor, Grace Kelley, and Jean Shrimpton at their "peak" will still appear beautiful to future generations, just as Botticelli's painting of *Venus* does to us today—but it's a pretty safe guess that Marilyn Monroe will be seen as a self-made sensation and Twiggy will simply look bizarre. (Without a doubt, if we could study a few pictures of Esther and Bathsheba right now, their beauty would stand the test of time amazingly well, too.)

As to what role this upper level of uncommon beauty plays in society, or for what purposes God chooses to create it, I'll leave that to learned philosophers, historians, sociologists, and theologians to debate. That we all recognize it when we see it is an intriguing, seemingly universal human phenomenon.[1] Even more amazing, however, isn't that God occasionally creates this kind of extraordinary beauty in a few exceptional women, but that He can make our hearts truly beautiful, as well. It's here, in the hidden places of our innermost beings, that His beauty powerfully exerts its most profound influence.

Hidden Beauty

In my life, I've seen countless attractive women. Of these, only a few were practically perfect. Their beauty was easy to identify. Whether walking down the street, sitting in a restaurant, posing in a magazine, or acting in a movie, such women are recognized immediately by almost everyone in our society. But there's a different kind of beauty—a genuine inner beauty of the heart—that is far more difficult to see.

Of all of the women I've encountered over the years, I remember only three who were extraordinarily beautiful in this way. I'm convinced that I would never have seen their beauty, if the Holy Spirit hadn't prompted me to look again: by today's cultural standards, none of these ladies would rank above a 2, let alone a 10! Yet they were so incredibly beautiful it brought tears to my eyes to behold them.

This isn't to say that women who are young or pleasing to look at can't be beautiful, too. They can. It's just that, in my experience, I've discovered that the most beautiful women I've seen were broken of their dependence on external appearances before the Lord's beauty was fully manifested.

One of these women, Corrie Ten Boom, was teaching from a podium when I first saw her. As she spoke, I couldn't take my eyes off her. Short, stout, and silver-haired, I noticed little else about Corrie other than her lively eyes and gentle smile. Oh, how she glowed! It didn't matter one iota that she wore her hair in a rather large, plain, nondescript bun on top of her head, or that she was attired in the clothing of an old-fashioned European grandmother: I'll never forget Corrie's welcoming, humble appearance. She was beautiful where it *really* counted—deep inside the hidden places of her heart.

Myrna Mosies is another woman who comes to my mind when I think about the kind of remarkable beauty the world usually misses but the Lord always sees. She was in her sixties when I first met her in 1971, shortly after I began following Jesus.

To be honest with you, Myrna was like many other Christian women I've known since then. Dedicated, kind, patient, and sweet-natured, she didn't wear much makeup and avoided fancy clothes while faithfully serving the church as our pastor's wife. But it wasn't until I saw her many years later, after we had moved away from Michigan and her husband went to be with the Lord, that I first witnessed the full brightness of Myrna's beauty bursting forth from her countenance, unhindered by the cares of this world.

Confined to a wheelchair after suffering a stroke, Myrna could no longer speak when I finally saw her again at my sister's wedding—she used her eyes to communicate instead. I can't describe exactly what I saw when I looked at Myrna then. She was shining, and she shone in such a way that I was overcome with tear-soaked joy, happily shaken by the sudden understanding that heaven wasn't very far from where we were sitting. Jesus touched me in a unique way through Myrna that day, with a spectacular kind of supernatural beauty I haven't encountered since.

There's one more woman whose beauty is so well disguised I doubt most people see it. I don't even know her name—she was being interviewed by a television crew when I caught my first glimpse of her. Yet, of all of the women I've ever seen or met, she displayed the rarest form of beauty.

I was getting ready in my hotel room for a speaking engagement. A national news station was playing in the background as I hurriedly tugged up my pantyhose and raced around searching for a lost earring. As I paused to think of what I needed to do next, I heard a woman quietly talking. Her peaceful voice drew me toward the television set as she recounted the experience of being burned over most of her body—including her head and face—in a terrible fire. Silently, I sat down on the bed and began listening.

At first, I was unprepared for the woman's extensive disfigurement. Her face was a mass of scars, knotted tissue, and splotchy skin; her nose had been reconstructed, but was still badly misshapen; she wore an awkward, ill-fitting wig because her own hair no longer grew. Everything most women rely on to look publicly presentable had been taken away from her in one brief, searing, tragic moment. Moreover, her appearance now, many months later, was actually frightening. *What must it be like to have a face like that,* I thought, *to utterly lose the way one has always looked?*

It took me a minute to look beyond the woman's injury and watch for her personality instead. Soon, I began to closely focus my attention only on her eyes. I noticed they were sparkling and bright!

There was no trace of self-pity in the woman's speech or demeanor. Instead, she sat with calm dignity before the camera as she shared about how Christ's love, and nothing else, was enabling her to move beyond the specter of her scars. "After all, wasn't He rejected, too?" I remember her asking. "Isn't Jesus also well-acquainted with suffering?"

With gentleness and strength, this woman courageously shared her story before an audience of millions. Tears welled up in my eyes as the beauty of the Lord made its indelible mark on me once more. Again, it wasn't merely sentiment or sympathy I was feeling, but encouragement—the deep, unshakable assurance of God's truth made real in a seemingly upside-down world. In this one woman, I saw Jesus: alive, resurrected, and gloriously triumphant. And He had won the victory.

The Image of Beauty

In the image of our beloved Savior, we find rest from the pressures of the world and are set free from the tyranny of today's beauty expectations. Through Jesus, our hearts are mysteriously and marvelously changed as the Holy Spirit breathes life, love, and liberty into the dry bones of our beings, fulfilling the promise we find in Ezekiel:

> I will give you a new heart and put a new spirit in you; I will remove from you your heart of stone and give you a heart of flesh.[2]

Transformed. Renewed. Born again. Forgiven. Accepted. Baptized unto Christ's death that we might live with Him in eternity. We've heard of these things many times before, but what do they have to do with beauty?

Everything. If we continually worry about the way we look or what we're wearing, focus too much on our weight and whether or not to go on a diet, berate our appearance while criticizing the appearances of others, compare ourselves to one another as we compete against our closest friends, get hung up on working out after feeling guilty for pigging out, and take pride in our "successes" after becoming depressed over any "failures" in this area, haven't we somehow forgotten something?

You bet we have. Until we are broken of our dependence on our own self-images, we cannot fully embrace the image of God in ourselves or each other. According to Dr. Paul Brand, a surgeon who has spent his life pioneering treatments for leprosy and performing reconstructive surgery on disabled patients, Jesus has already taught us this wonderful lesson: the kind of beauty the world values most is worthless in comparison to the holy magnificence of God's great glory dwelling within us.

Dr. Brand writes:

> God reproduces and lives out His image in millions of ordinary people like us. It is a supreme mystery.
>
> We are called to bear that image as a Body because any one of us taken individually would present an incomplete image, one partly false and always distorted, like a single glass chip hacked away from a mirror. But collectively, in all our diversity, we can come together as a community of believers to restore the image of God in the world.
>
> For a pattern to follow, we need only look back at Jesus, that divine image seared into our consciousness. The surprising qualities he showed—humility, servanthood, love—become the model for His Body also. No longer must we struggle to build up our own images, to prove ourselves. Rather, we can focus our lives on showing forth His image. And what counts for great success in popular culture—strength, intelligence, wealth, beauty, power—means little to that image. . . .
>
> The beautiful, the strong, the politically powerful, and the rich do not easily represent God's image. Rather, His spirit shines most brightly through the frailty of the weak, the impotence of the poor, the deformity of the hunchback. Even as bodies are broken, His image can grow brighter. . . .
>
> I do not say that a Miss Universe or a handsome Olympian can never show forth the love and power of God,

but I do believe that such a person is, in some ways, at a disadvantage. Talent, a pleasing physical appearance, and the adulation of crowds tend to shove aside the qualities of humility and love that Christ demands of those who would bear His image. . . .

When we join His Body, it is the image of God Himself we must find, not our own. We find it not by proving ourselves, but by releasing that desperate dependence on our own self-images in favor of taking on His own glorious image. . . . It is His glory we take on, not our own. The cost may increase for those with wealth, physical attraction, and security. But for all of us, the reward is the same: a chance not to be judged for what we are but for what Christ is. When God looks upon us He sees His beloved Son.[3]

As strange as it may seem to us, you and I are God's image-bearers here on earth—whether we're a size two or a size 20. We belong to Him, not to ourselves. As His Body, we're collectively called to make Him visible, in flesh and bone, before a watching world.

Where Beauty Begins

How can this be? I really don't know. Nobody does, in fact. What we *do* know, though, is that the Spirit of God enters our lives and absolutely changes us when we receive Jesus into our hearts. Afterwards, we're never the same again.

My favorite illustration of this experience is in a book by C. S. Lewis called *That Hideous Strength.* Jane is a thoroughly contemporary woman—educated, independent, and highly opinionated. Before becoming converted, she is intellectually detached from her own femininity and, in her mind, its relationship to servility, male dominance—

and to her husband, Mark. But the Lord has a better plan for Jane's life.

As her heart begins to open up to God after several long conversations with a Christian leader in her community named the Director, Jane receives an unexpected visit from the Holy Spirit. Here's how Lewis describes the encounter:

> Jane had gone into the garden to think. She accepted what the Director had said, yet it seemed to her nonsensical. His comparison between Mark's love and God's (since apparently there was a God) struck her nascent spirituality as indecent and irreverent. "Religion" ought to mean a realm in which her haunting female fear of being treated as a thing, an object of barter and desire and possession, would be set permanently at rest and what she called her "true self" would soar upwards and expand in some freer and purer world. For still she thought that "Religion" was a kind of exhalation or a cloud of incense, something streaming up from specially gifted souls toward a receptive heaven. . . . Supposing one were a thing after all—a thing designed and invented by Someone Else and valued for qualitites different from what one had decided to regard as one's true self? Supposing all those people who, from the bachelor uncles down to Mark and Mother Dimble, had infuriatingly found her sweet and fresh when she wanted them to find her also interesting and important, had all along been simply right and perceived the sort of thing she was? Supposing [God] on this subject agreed with them and not with her? For one moment she had a ridiculous and scorching vision of a world in which God Himself would never understand, never take her with full seriousness. Then, at one particular corner of the gooseberry patch, the change came.
>
> What awaited her there was serious to the degree of sorrow and beyond. There was no form or sound. The mould under the bushes, the moss on the path, and the little brick border were not visibly changed. But they were changed. A

boundary had been crossed. She had come into a world, or into a Person, or into the presence of a Person. Something expectant, patient, inexorable, met her with no veil or protection between. . . . This demand which now pressed upon her was not, even by analogy, like any other demand. It was the origin of all right demands and contained them. In its light you could understand them; but from them you could know nothing of it. There was nothing, and never had been anything, like this. And now there was nothing except this. Yet also, everything had been like this; only by being like this had anything existed. In this height and depth and breadth the little idea of herself which she had hitherto called me dropped down and vanished, unfluttering, into bottomless distance, like a bird in space without air. The name me was the name of a being whose existence she had never suspected, a being that did not yet fully exist but which was demanded. It was a person (not the person she had thought), yet also a thing, a made thing, made to please Another and in Him to please all others, a thing being made at this very moment, without its choice, in a shape it had never dreamed of. And the making went on amidst a kind of splendor or sorrow or both, whereof she could not tell whether it was in the molding hands or in the kneaded lump. . . .

To be aware of this and to know that it had already gone made one single experience. It was revealed only in its departure. The largest thing that had ever happened to her had, apparently, found room for itself in a moment of time too short to be called time at all. Her hand closed on nothing but a memory. And as it closed, without an instant's pause, the voices of those who have not joy rose howling and chattering from every corner of her being.

"Take care. Draw back. Keep your head. Don't commit yourself," they said. And then more subtly, from another quarter, "You have had a religious experience. This is very interesting. Not everyone does. How much better you will now understand the Seventeenth-Century poets!" Or from a third direction, more sweetly, "Go on. Try to get it again. It will please the Director."

But her defenses had been captured and these counter-attacks were unsuccessful.[4]

For Jane, this moment was a clear, historic point of departure from the woman she had previously been. For each of us, although becoming a new creation happens in its own unique way, our experience of conversion is also strikingly similar: Christ's beauty is birthed in our hearts as the old self dies and we receive our new identity in Him. As we accept our dependence upon God—our *creatureliness*—we relinquish our own god-like presumptions, and gladly submit ourselves to being reshaped according to the image of Jesus Christ through the power of the Holy Spirit.

From this starting point of complete openness and vulnerability before our heavenly Father, we are transformed into the likeness of His Son. *Satan hates this.* He'll try anything to destroy Christ's image within us and distract us from our primary calling—loving and serving the Lord with our whole hearts, in the joy and freedom of the Holy Spirit.

I'm convinced that beauty issues have become one of the enemy's principle means of attack against the image of Christ we bear. We must actively resist being manipulated and influenced, standing firm against the powers and principalities which plant seeds of despair and doubt in our minds about our true identity in Christ.

The next time you go to the grocery store or pharmacy, try something unusual. Walk over to the magazine rack and stand in front of the women's section without looking closely at any of the covers. Closing your eyes for a moment, pray that you'll be able to spiritually discern what is going on in the pictures when you open your eyes again. Ask God for wisdom and understanding. You might even want to imagine that you've never seen these kind of magazines before—in a sense, it may be as if you really *are* seeing them accurately for the first time!

Just as we need to become more sensitive to the Holy Spirit in order to see what the Lord's beauty *is*, we must also learn to grow in our ability to discern what it *isn't.* You may have already had plenty of practice with this, or it may be an entirely new experience to you. Don't be surprised if you feel a little defensive about doing this exercise. After all, you've been bombarded by false imitations of the real thing on a daily basis, from almost every direction imaginable, since you were a little girl. Go ahead and do it anyway.

Now, open your eyes.

Seeing and Believing

As we develop discernment about beauty and are broken of our dependence upon appearances, mind-boggling things start to happen. In my own life, it's meant looking in the mirror more often without reacting with admiration or anxiety, but with acceptance. When I eat or exercise, I know I can respectfully care for my body without punishing it. My husband's opinion of the way I look no longer makes or breaks my day, though I still enjoy pleasing him. And, best of all, I'm more frequently forgetting how I look as I increasingly remember to look for Christ's image in the lives of others.

Isn't it good to know that in Jesus "we live and move and have our being"?[5] That we don't have to prove our worth to God by who we are and how we look and what we do? Getting this truth deep down inside our hearts enlarges our capacity to love Jesus more joyfully in all of life's circumstances—to be the women Christ calls us to be rather than who our culture or other people expect us to be.

Today's emphasis on physical beauty distorts and diminishes this calling. The frustration we feel when we buy into cultural images of beauty is a natural response to what happens when we become disconnected from the real source of our beauty: the image of Christ dwelling inside us. Feeling perpetually inadequate or self-conscious isn't how our Creator intends us to live. Instead, it's an internal warning mechanism if we choose to heed it.

Thankfully, we can ask God to shatter the molds that have previously shaped us:

> . . . by God's mercy to offer your very selves to him: a living sacrifice, dedicated and fit for his acceptance, the worship offered by mind and heart. Adapt yourselves no longer to the pattern of this present world, but let your minds be remade and your whole nature thus transformed. Then you will be able to discern the will of God, and know what is good, acceptable, and perfect.[6]

In fulfilling this command, we become part of a rich legacy that affirms our calling as Christians and identity as women. L'Abri director Dick Keyes expresses it this way: "God's salvation restores men and women to the true image of God, the original." He also explains:

Being conformed to something less than the image of God is wrong for two reasons. First it is wrong because the old mold is rebellion against God and involves a refusal to obey Him. Second, no other mold is big enough or rich enough to allow our individuality to grow within it. All other molds are smaller than the one you were made for. Only God the Creator is great enough to be our final point of integration, the one whose character we shape ourselves around. . . . The person seeking her identity through other people, whether it be from a particular group or the mass of humanity, is trapped in unreality. She will agonize over her image, her speech, her personal appearance, all the while hating herself for caring so much about what everybody else thinks. . . .

Whatever stands in the way of the image of God must be put off—whether it be a habit, an attitude, an idea, or any of the social molds we have just mentioned. To grow as a Christian we must be weaned from the things that are less than God which have come to take the place of God in us.[7]

"If you are a Christian," Keyes concludes, "your final environment is a world whose Creator forgives, accepts, and loves you in all your uniqueness. God not only loves you in this way, but he wants you to always be aware of it. He wants you to have that confidence and to live in it."[8]

Our confidence is based, then, not on our own understanding of who we are, but on the truth of God's promise: "The secret is this: Christ in you, the hope of a glory to come."[9] Even if we can't quite comprehend this wonderful reality yet, we can ask the Lord to help us believe it.

By God's grace, we can reject counterfeit images of beauty, breaking the molds that bind us and finding healing for our hearts. Let's not settle for anything less than the best: a real and lasting beauty wrought deep within us by God's own hand.

Action Plan

A Place to Begin

Changing from the outside in is very difficult, if not impossible. We can try to change, to give up our fascination and/or compulsion towards the beauty culture. We may be able to change for a while, but we invariably slip back into old patterns and ways unless we are changed from the inside out. And how do we change that way?

By becoming a Christian and letting Jesus Christ do the work.

• If you want to know more about how to become a Christian or would like to enter into a deeper relationship with Jesus, you don't have to wait to talk with an "expert" or read a recent book on the subject of salvation before getting started. It is not difficult to receive Jesus Christ as your Savior. To do so you must first confess your need of a Savior. Then believe that Jesus Christ is the Son of God and that He died to provide a perfect salvation for you. Last of all, ask Him to wash away all your sin and make you His child forever.

• In addition, ask the Lord to lead you to someone who can offer you spiritual direction and practical support, and begin actively looking for Christian fellowship. Attend a regular Bible study in addition to weekly services. As you grow in your understanding of the Bible, passages that formerly seemed incomprehensible will suddenly appear clearer. Stay hungry for the nourishment that God's Word alone can provide.

• Read through the following Scriptures to get a clear picture of the new life of faith you will receive after being born into God's family:

John 3:1-21
Romans 5:1-11
Ephesians 1:3-13, 2:4-8
Colossians 1:21-23

• Once we have become a child of God and fully understand our value to Him, we will be able to stop and consider who we are and where we are going. Then we can make decisions about the whole beauty issue from the standpoint of what matters in eternity. This realization will transform our outlook and clarify our calling.

❧ *Focus Questions* ❧

1. Considering beauty from a spiritual vantage point, who are the most beautiful women you know? What strikes you most about them? How has their beauty deepened your own understanding of beauty?

2. Name some of the barriers that affect people's ability to see God's image clearly in themselves and others. When you see people, what do you notice first about them?

3. Is it difficult for you to accept God's unconditional love for you? If so, what walls need to come down in your life for you to fully embrace Him?

Nine

Adornments of the Heart

*Take from us, O God, all pride and vanity, all boasting
and forwardness, and give us the true courage that
shows itself by gentleness; the true wisdom that shows
itself by simplicity; and the true power that shows itself by
modesty; through Jesus Christ our Lord.*

— *Charles Kingsley, 1819-1875*

*Hold fast the faith which God has given you by His
Holy Spirit; it is the most precious treasure in this life,
and it contains in itself true happiness. Only seek by
watching and prayer more and more to be delivered from
all vanity and self-complacency, by which even the true
believer may be ensnared when he least expects it.
Let it be your chief aim to be more and more humble,
faithful, and quiet.*

— *From a letter written by a
German woman to George Mueller, 1827*

I like to read. Public and university libraries are my favorite city places, with the exception of riding the Westin Peachtree Plaza glass elevator, which soars some 60 stories up into the Atlanta skyline, or being at Fulton County Stadium when the Braves hit a home run.

When my daughters and sons were little, I went to the library to relax. It was quiet there, and I could sit for more than an hour without any interruptions. Our neighborhood library also served another purpose: the kids and I regularly went to story time and checked out children's books to read and enjoy at home. Some of these stories continue to remain close to my heart. Later, libraries became the place where I went to work if I needed additional information. While researching one project, upon reaching my limit of 99 books, I ended up carrying the stacks back and forth to the University of Nebraska circulation desk in a laundry basket. I doubt I'll ever do that again.

Now that I'm 40, when I'm not helping the kids with term papers or doing research for my writing, my husband and I visit libraries for fun. We scan magazines and newspapers, compare new titles, and consult reference works for upcoming presentations and speeches. These "dates," if not thrilling, are *free*, and our weekly outings are often fruitful.

During the summer of 1992, Dave and I jointly decided to read a science fiction thriller by Michael Crichton called *Jurassic Park*.

Now a blockbuster movie, it's about genetically cloned dinosaurs wreaking havoc on an island near Costa Rica. Drawn to the book for its what-if presentation of the possible effects of genetic engineering on creation, we took turns reading the text and discussing our reactions. A passage near the opening of Crichton's book immediately caught my attention:

> Mike Bowman whistled cheerfully as he drove the Land Rover through the Cabo Blanco Biological Reserve, on the west coast of Costa Rica. It was a beautiful morning in July, and the road before him was spectacular hugging the edge of the cliff, overlooking the jungle and the blue Pacific. According to the guidebooks, Cabo Blanco was unspoiled wilderness, almost a paradise. Seeing it now made Bowman feel as if the vacation was back on track.
>
> Bowman, a thirty-six-year-old real estate developer from Dallas, had come to Costa Rica with his wife and daughter for a two-week holiday. The trip had actually been his wife's idea; for weeks Ellen had filled his ear about the wonderful national parks of Costa Rica, and how good it would be for Tina to see them. Then, when they arrived, it turned out Ellen had an appointment to see a plastic surgeon in San Jose. That was the first Mike Bowman had heard about the inexpensive plastic surgery available in Costa Rica, and all the luxurious private clinics in San Jose.
>
> Of course they'd had a huge fight. Mike felt she'd lied to him, and she had. And he put his foot down about the plastic surgery business. Anyway, it was ridiculous, Ellen was only thirty, and she was a beautiful woman. She'd been Homecoming Queen her senior year at Rice, and that was not even ten years earlier. But Ellen tended to be insecure, and worried. And it seemed as if in recent years she had mostly worried about losing her looks. . . . Ellen got out a

compact and looked at herself in the mirror, pressing under her eyes. She sighed, and put the compact away. . . .

He parked the Land Rover in the shade of the palm trees that fringed the beach, and got out the box lunches. Ellen changed into her bathing suit, saying, "Honestly, I don't know how I'm going to get this weight off."

"You look great, hon." Actually, he felt she was too thin, but he had learned not to mention that.

Tina was already running down the beach.

"Don't forget your sunscreen," Ellen called.[1]

This, in a book written by a man, at the beginning of a male-oriented book! (Only one of the main characters is a woman—a young blonde scientist with a great body, beautiful face, and long legs.) Since the Bowmans never turn up again, these details are even more intriguing. Crichton could have chosen to say anything about Ellen Bowman, but writing as a Harvard graduate, ex-physician, best-selling author, and wealthy Californian involved in the movie industry, this is what he decided to say. Given the opportunity, I think many men would share a similar message: vanity is a turn-off. It makes looking good repulsive, and it leaves room in a woman's heart for nothing but herself. What a waste!

I finished the book, and so did Dave. Of the two of us, however, I was the only one who remembered (and copied) the passage about the Bowmans. Because, like it or not, there's a little bit of Ellen in every woman I know, including me.

False Promises, Lasting Truths

How do you spot a false god? A false god is a controlling factor in a person's life and usurps God's right to rulership. It can be anything, or anyone, we fix our attention and focus our minds upon.

False gods capture people's hearts and minds. Easy to identify in others' lives, they're often difficult to discern in our own. Popular jargon uses updated language to describe them—for example, addiction, codependency, enabling, and empowerment. But as Juliet said to Romeo, "A rose by any other name would smell as sweet," and new terms for false gods don't change their true identity. Sought after as a primary source of satisfaction or significance, a false god motivates one's mouth, directs one's eyes, and screens out any competing interests. Consequently, it gradually dominates a person's life.

Making a list of today's false gods isn't difficult. All it takes is a brief visit to any general bookstore or library.[2] By searching the racks and then tallying types of titles, you'll find out pretty quickly who and what they are: work, success, health and fitness, achievement, food and dieting, wealth, sex, romance, marriage and family, art, spiritual growth, home decorating and improvement, technology, politics, knowledge, comfort, power, fashion, sports, intimacy, travel, entertainment, inner happiness, beauty, fantasy, finance, and self-actualization.

These things offer greater personal pleasure and fulfillment, and most are enjoyable if kept in proper perspective.[3] But none ultimately fulfills our deepest longings and innermost need for love, joy, and peace.

In church on Sunday, the epistle verse read at the pulpit said: "Do not live for money; be content with what you have."[4] Words that could have been written this week. In the Book of Acts we're told, "All the Athenians and foreigners who lived there spent their time doing nothing but talking about and listening to the latest ideas"[5]—an appropriate description of practically every talk show on television today. When offered the kingdoms of this world, Jesus answered: "You shall worship the Lord your God and Him alone shall you serve."[6] It's obvious that Satan's thirst for souls hasn't changed in the least: the devil still tempts Christ's followers today.

Just as none of these things have changed, neither has the human propensity for serving idols.[7] A false god can attract and trap any of us no matter how long we've known the Lord and won't surrender its grip on our minds and hearts without putting up a fight. Prayers and biblical phrases—although vitally essential—are not a sufficient rebuke. To denounce a false god and destroy its power, we must also rebuke it with our lives.

Setting Our Sights with a Single Mind

Today's image cult creates an almost irresistible focus on physical attractiveness, body shape, sexuality, and clothing styles. The Word of God gives us a clear alternative: "Seek first the kingdom of God and His righteousness."[8] Making this commandment our life's goal demonstrates who we belong to and what we're here for as true children of our King. But in practical terms, how do we actually *do* it?

"We are called to seek the kingdom by bearing witness to the kingdom," says theologian Dr. R. C. Sproul. He further explains:

> We are to seek to show the world what the kingdom of God looks like. For the kingdom to come on earth as it is in

heaven means that loyal children of the King do the King's will here and now. We bear witness to God's kingdom by serving God's King.

This is the will of God. This is what pleases Him. There is a reason why Jesus links the coming of the kingdom with the doing of the will of God. "Your kingdom come. Your will be done," belong together. They are two sides of the same coin. The kingdom comes on earth where God's will is done on earth. The conclusion we reach is this: The great overarching goal of the Christian life is *obedience to the King.* And He is pleased when we obey.[9]

Seeking the kingdom means surrendering "every proud and lofty thing that sets itself up against the (true) knowledge of God."[10] It means keeping our eyes on Jesus and doing what is right in God's sight. None of us can do this perfectly. That's part of the reason God became one of us—people had already tried to be righteous and had failed. This central focus of loving, honoring, and serving our King, placing Jesus in the highest place in our hearts, and connecting what we think and say and do to the reality of His presence in our lives, powerfully rebukes the enemy and renounces the false gods of our age.

But seeking God's Kingdom does much more: it also brings us real happiness and freedom, removing the inner instability and insecurity that result from having divided loyalties and a double mind.[11] When we desire God and seek Him wholeheartedly, we come home. Concerning this, George MacDonald once wrote:

> Christ is the way out and the way in; the way from slavery, conscious or unconscious, into liberty; the way from the unhomeliness of things to the home we desire but do not know; the way from the stormy skirts of the Father's garments to the peace of His bosom.[12]

Again Jesus promises that "Whoever finds his [lower] life will lose [the higher life], and whoever loses his [lower] life on My account will find the [higher] life."[13] We can't have it both ways—and when we try to, we end up miserable or desperate. Thank God for the glory of His Kingdom and the homeliness of His righteousness!

Bearing Witness

As a woman, I resist different temptations than my husband does, and subsequently bear witness to God's Kingdom in a different way. Without giving out details, I'd say the things Dave deals with are pretty typical for a 44-year-old man. Conversely, much of what God is currently working on in my life isn't unusual for a woman my age, either.

In spite of these differences—which at times provoke each of us to take pride in our own "safe" positions—we walk a common road. Our calling, while expressed uniquely, is nevertheless the same: to love God with all our hearts and with all our souls and with all our minds, and to love our neighbors as ourselves.[14]

My husband and I can't obey this commandment *for, through,* or *because of* one another. It's strictly a one-on-one responsibility between God and Dave, and God and me. As we walk with the Lord moment by moment, the Holy Spirit intimately leads, guides, and makes Jesus known to each of us. He also convicts us of sin—but He doesn't convict me of Dave's sin and then charge me with setting him right again, or vice versa.

Let's say that I'm feeling fat and can't keep my mind

off my weight. All day long, I think about food—avoiding food, eating certain kinds of foods, cooking diet dinners, feeling ashamed if I overeat, feeling great if I don't. Food has become my daily focus, even though I'm trying to lose weight with God's help and for His glory. I exercise, shop correctly, and snack on baby carrots. Every time we go out to eat, I ask the waitress or counter person about numbers of calories and fat grams, complaining about Diet Coke tasting like chemicals. While getting dressed in front of my husband, I point out my burgeoning waistline and inquire about his opinion of my wide behind. Beyond all of this, I also talk to Dave constantly about this struggle because I think he should be sharing this burden.

You tell me: is this kind of behavior attractive to my husband? Is it beneficial for both of us to become involved with my false god? Beyond asking for prayer and support, why would I expect Dave to take care of the problem? It's my responsibility, not Dave's, and when I ask him to inappropriately get involved with managing a false god I'm facing, he may end up serving it, too. My idolatry is up to me to handle.

For too long, I looked to the false gods of my culture to tell me how to make myself more beautiful. I've concentrated more on pleasing people than pleasing God, and I've listened to all kinds of lies regarding beauty and femininity. Making me unhappy and unattractive, vanity kept me captivated by my own image in the mirror, and blocked the view of Christ's image in myself and others. Since convicting me of this, the Holy Spirit is also teaching me what to do about it without seeking anyone else's affirmation or approval. Believe me, this has been a big relief for both Dave and me!

Here, in the context of our closest relationships, faithfully bearing witness to the Kingdom begins. Whether married or single, the way we interact and react to people around us reflects what, and whom, we serve.

No More Manipulation

The following passage, written by an actress named Arlene Dahl, describes the attitude about beauty I grew up believing—an attitude that continues to captivate many women today. From a biblical standpoint, it stands in stark contrast to the qualities the New Testament calls Christians to seek:

> All truly feminine women have one basic quality in common. They like men. Male company can make a woman feel warm and content, glamorous and exuberant, interested, and interesting.
>
> Men have a sixth sense about women. They respond to us in exactly the same degree that we respond to them. A feminine woman makes a man feel important. Instinctively, she works at pleasing him. When she likes a man and it's returned, she lights up from inside and the glow shines through her eyes and smile. When he speaks to her, she listens with rapt attention to every word. George Hamilton believes that femininity is the most appealing quality in a woman. "She can get whatever she wants, not by being forceful, but by being feminine. A woman is often like a strip of film—obliterated, insignificant—until a man puts the light behind her."[15]

This isn't femininity. It's manipulation! It's a seductive approach to womanliness that feeds on others to validate and affirm one's identity—a key component of idolatry's grip in any form. Jesus is the light that brightens my life, not men. As a Christian woman, I refuse to believe this myth about beauty any longer.

If not this, then what *do* we do about our appearance in relation to seeking the Kingdom first—especially as it relates to men? This is what I've started doing: *learning how to be beautiful in a whole new context as God deals with my fear of rejection and need for approval from others.* As I ask Jesus for freedom and wisdom in my life, I've been astounded at all the things I've needed to change. But it's been an exhilarating, rather than a burdensome, process. Getting rid of all that excess baggage is a huge relief!

After vacationing with my sister last summer and studying a number of classic Christian texts, I began thinking more about how women's appearances affect men, including my own. I especially noticed the way women "adorn themselves" in church-related settings and understood my motivations better in this regard. Significantly toning down my makeup, I also started to dress differently. And I stopped worrying about my weight.

At first, these changes felt uncomfortable and left a void in my life. I'd grown so accustomed to relying on my appearance to communicate who I was that it seemed to be a part of me instead of a temporary tent for my spirit. With less makeup and other adornments, I felt less self-assured, somewhat unsteady, even a little shy. But as the weeks rolled by, I actually started enjoying silently serving Jesus in this way.

That's when it struck me: what if *all* women started doing this? I quizzed a number of male friends and family members, asking them, "Would you find it easier not to look at the women you work with if they wore simpler styles, little jewelry, and less makeup?" They all nodded an emphatic yes.

It's a vicious cycle: since men are used to women doing everything in their power to enhance their appearance, most expect women to engage in manipulative beauty behaviors. Consequently, boys in the high school youth group tend not to notice girls who are beautiful on the inside *and* plain or overweight on the outside: they go for the "lookers" instead. Pretty girls marry faster than "ordinary" ones; husbands with attractive wives feel proud to be seen with them. This is tragic, isn't it? Our culture hasn't only affected women, it has affected men deeply, too, and everyone's suffering as a result.

What's needed today is the far-reaching realization that many of today's beliefs and attitudes about beauty fit our culture, not Scripture. Men and women alike need to repent for serving the false gods associated with physical attractiveness and personal appearance. In humility, we need to ask God's forgiveness, and move toward a higher calling.

Dressing Our Hearts

Modesty is more than covering the body: it's also an attitude of guarding one's heart, mind, soul, and spirit out of love and devotion for Jesus Christ. It's God's solution to the poison of vanity and pride—a holy antidote to our destructive bent toward dependence on outward appearances. Practicing this virtue protects us from harm.

As Paul wrote to Timothy:

> I want men everywhere to lift up holy hands in prayer, without anger or disputing. I also want women to dress modestly, with decency and propriety, not with braided hair or gold or pearls or expensive clothes, but with good deeds, appropriate for women who profess to worship God.[16]

Our culture's brand of femininity—using your looks to get a man (or keep your husband) any way you can—isn't our King's. To be beautiful for Jesus, we must look to Him for affirmation regarding who we are and offer our lives to Him in love. Seeking His kingdom and right way of living before everything else signals others that we're not "available"—*we belong to God.* Our eyes are no longer glued to watching ourselves or our culture, but turned toward our Lord.

It's helpful to remember this first thing every morning. Upon waking up, we can choose what and whom to set our minds upon: thanking God for His indwelling presence, why not put on the spiritual armor of battle and clothing of Christ before even getting out of bed?[17] Memorizing and meditating upon the Word of God—including the Lord's Prayer, 23rd Psalm, and fruit of the Holy Spirit[18]—clears our thinking and restores our sight.

Specifics concerning what each of us do or don't do about hair, makeup, and clothing aren't important. Listen to the Lord as you ask Him to teach you what you need to change. Pray for wisdom.[19] As you get dressed and apply your makeup, avoid adornments that distract your attention—and the attention of others—from Christ. Walk through everyday interactions knowing your words and actions matter to the Master because He *loves* you and is jealous for your affection. Adorn your heart for Him.

Jesus promises to supply your every need, no matter how trifling or small it may seem.[20] In surrendering our dependence on outward appearances, we begin to wear the raiment of our King.

Action Plan

Moving On

Before we even climb out of bed in the morning, we need to put on the armor of God. It's easier for me to remember if I start at the top of my head and work my way down. Then, when I'm fully clothed in His armor, I ask the Lord to equip me with a sword and shield.

Here's my list starting from the head down:

The armor of God:
    helmet of salvation
    breastplate of righteousness
    belt of truth
    feet fitted with the readiness that comes from
    the gospel of *peace*
    sword of the Spirit: the Word of God
    shield of faith

The clothing of Christ:
    compassion
    kindness
    humility
    gentleness
    patience

The fruit of the Spirit:
  love
  joy
  peace
  patience
  kindness
  goodness
  faithfulness
  gentleness
  self-control

• Beyond mentally "putting on" this clothing of God (Ephesians 6:10-20) and asking for the fruit, only the Holy Spirit can provide (Galations 5:22,23), it is also helpful to memorize the Lord's Prayer (Matthew 6:9-13) and the 23rd Psalm. Having God's Word in our hearts is absolutely essential to strengthening our spirits, clearing our thinking, and restoring our sight.

• Prepare a list of other pertinent passages and keep them handy to use both offensively and defensively—as needed. Remember: Scripture is meant to be used frequently, along with praying in the Spirit (Ephesians 6:18).

• Ask the Lord what you need to change and don't worry about specifics concerning your hair, makeup, or clothing. As you dress each morning, concentrate on adorning your heart for Him.

• Wait on the Lord, choosing to let go of your anxieties—including the need to look and be perfect. If possible, find a quiet place to communicate with Jesus, but if you can't, then pray while doing the dishes, driving to work, or rocking the baby to sleep. This is the source that provides us with hidden strength that can't be taken from us.

• Don't be surprised if you discover—as I have—how many behaviors and thought patterns need changing. Change is a process, so don't be discouraged by momentary setbacks or slip-ups as you strive to overcome today's image cult. Sometimes, it's good to laugh about this unavoidable predicament; otherwise, we take ourselves far too seriously for our own good. At other times, confession and repentance offer the only possible solution for change.

• Ask the Holy Spirit to heal you of the hurts you've already received at the hands of today's beauty culture. Whether or not you've given into the pressure to starve yourself, to have plastic surgery, or to indulge in expensive cosmetics and clothes, we all need the Lord's healing touch.

🌱 *Focus Questions* 🌿

1. What is vanity? How is it expressed most in your life?
2. In your opinion, why do you think women are vulnerable to using their appearance to manipulate men?
3. In what ways are women harmed by their own lack of modesty? By today's trends in clothing design?

Ten

Bondage to Beauty or Breaking Free?

*The true way to be humble is not to stoop until you are
smaller than yourself, but to stand at your real height
against some higher nature that will show you what the
real smallness of your greatness is.*

—— *Phillips Brooks, 1872*

*A man is in bondage to whatever he cannot part with
that is less than himself.*

—— *George MacDonald, 1824-1905*

*J*esus *rarely comes where we expect Him,"* says Oswald Chambers in *My Utmost for His Highest.* "He appears where we least expect Him, and always in the most illogical connections."[1]

A number of years ago, one of these "illogical connections" happened to me. Sponsored by the hospital where I worked, a continuing education workshop on human sexuality promised to be especially interesting because it was going to be taught by a celibate woman—Sister Mary Christelle Macaluso, a professor at Sacred Heart College in Omaha. At first, I admit, I was a little skeptical about signing up. (A *nun* teaching about sex? What could *she* possibly know?) I went ahead and registered, mostly out of curiosity, but also because it's difficult to find this subject presented from a uniquely Christian perspective.

Happily, the eight hours I spent with Sister Macaluso were among the most memorable I've experienced with an educator. Blessed with an incredible sense of humor, she had every participant eagerly involved in her topic from the first sentence, caught up in a refreshing blend of mirth and merriment rarely seen in a professional setting. Using storytelling, cartoons, short films, and traditional wisdom, Sister Mary Christelle knew her subject well, emphasizing that whether single or married, we're *all* sexual beings according to God's design—a fact well worth celebrating with a certain amount of hilarity as well as seriousness.

One of the films shown that day left an indelible impression on me. Its sole subject was a baby about 14 months of age, dressed only in a diaper. The child busily engaged in typical toddler things: climbing up the side of a sofa, giggling and squirming, rolling on a carpet, making funny faces, playfully pushing a ball around, smiling at the camera, sucking on each toe. There was no narration whatsoever until the very last moment. As the film ends, the child peers into the camera, and an announcer simply says, *"You."*

This engaging portrayal of a one-year-old's exuberant excitement reminds us of our own inner beauty, gently provoking each viewer to reflect on his or her earliest life experiences: the joy of each fresh discovery, the mastery of a new movement, the bright realities of one's *here and now.* It also reminded me of life before I became so conscious of myself: no clothing concerns, no cosmetics to apply, no complicated hairstyles to do, no climbing on the scales from one morning to the next—just a tremendous freedom to *be,* without getting all wound up inside about all sorts of stuff that doesn't really matter.

In observing the simplicity of this baby, I saw how complicated I'd become. That's when God surprised me. In a silent whisper, it was as if I could hear Him say, "I love you, Debra, not for what you *look* like but for who you *are* in My Son. Did not the Lord your Maker create you well? Did I not fashion every inch of you the way *I* intended you to be? Why do you worry so much about all these things? *I love you!"*

Turning Turkeys into Eagles

Kids, of course, don't worry about these things. What they do instead is *live*—energetically, expressively, enthusiastically—without comparing. Children aren't innocent or unselfish creatures, yet Jesus wants us to become more like them, in order to enter His kingdom.[2]

"Our true nature is to be a child of the Father," declares author and physician Dr. John White. "As we relate to Him on a daily basis, something within us will develop more and more. *We will become different persons.* Formerly turkeys, we will become eagles. Our wings will grow, our necks shorten, our wattles disappear. Isaiah told us that placing our hope in God would result in renewed strength. We would run effortlessly, soar on eagle wings."[3]

I don't know about you, but I'm tired of feeling like a turkey when it comes to chasing after impossible beauty ideals. I'd *much* prefer to be soaring on eagle's wings (and to be honest, these wattles have been really getting to me lately). *I'm ready for a change, but the change I'm looking for can't come from me*—it can only come from turning toward my heavenly Father as the one sure source of my identity.

As adults, we often question where kids get all their energy. My guess is that much of the fatigue we grown-ups feel has nothing to do with God's will or growing older: it's partially the result of running our own non-stop marathon to "look and feel our best" day in and day out. (At times, I've been so burned out from trying to keep up that Isaiah's words started to sound like a totally foreign concept to me.)

If we're feeling worn-out just thinking about our

clothes, weight, and appearance, it's a sure sign that we're missing the mark in our walk with Jesus. Insecurity, restlessness, vanity, anxiety, envy, and discontentment are all part of the package deal when it comes to serving beauty. These things can't possibly make us happy—in fact, they're guaranteed to make us totally miserable! But Jesus doesn't leave us here. Opening His arms wide, He sees our hurting hearts, and calls: "Come unto me." The promise found in Isaiah is true: those who hope in the Lord will renew their strength as they find sanctuary in God's presence.[4]

The peace and rest we desire may not happen instantly. In fact, the release we seek may come slowly, as we continue to "press on toward the goal to win the prize for which God has called us heavenward in Christ Jesus."[5] In the meantime, says John White:

> Give yourself a break. Expand your wings and soar! You can change. Permanently. For the better. From within. You can repent. Or, if you repented long ago, you can move into a life of ongoing repentance. . . .
>
> God Himself has paid the price. He will be glad to initiate the process, enter your life, and impart his own nature to you. If he entered long ago, he can now change His relationship to you radically. How incredible the fact may appear, God yearns for intimacy with you. And he wants you to respond.
>
> There is a price, of course. There was for God, and there will be for you. The price is to face the truth—primarily the truth about yourself, your sin, and your helplessness to change matters. It's humiliating, but then, a little bit of humility never hurt anybody. In fact it heals. And in any case, who are you or I to keep the Creator of the universe waiting?[6]

When I hear words such as these, initially I feel slightly

silly—silly about the amount of time, energy, and effort I waste on the nonessentials in life. Then I sigh in relief. As the world's heaviness drops from my shoulders, I start to grin and want to shout: *God loves me! He accepts me exactly as I am! I'm complete in Him!*

Shepherd of My...

I was a Christian for almost 20 years before I began determinedly laying down my beauty-related fears and worries. Somehow, my need for spiritual release in this area escaped my attention altogether—even though I constantly worried about my weight, tried to impress people by the way I looked, and was hooked on comparing myself to other women. When I looked at my sisters in Christ, the first things I noticed about them tended to be their size, facial attractiveness, hairstyle, clothes, and jewelry, instead of their personhood. By concentrating on women's appearances, I missed the most important thing: the reflection of God's image displayed in one-of-a-kind style.

I used to associate idolatry with huge marble statues of Greco-Roman goddesses, not photos of models on billboards and in magazines. Yet, in focusing my thoughts and energy on conforming to these images, I wasn't serving God at all—I was bowing to the idols of my culture.[7] Although I looked to Jesus as the Shepherd of my heart and soul, it didn't strike me as being important for Him to be Shepherd of my *face* and *body*, too.

Then, God began to heal a few of my blind spots and restore my sight. First, I saw how desperately I needed Him to turn my thinking around to conform to His truth: I needed some remaking and reshaping at the inner-most center of my identity. Second, I required deliverance from the lies I'd been told about beauty and its relationship to femininity through the truth of God's Word. Third, I realized how deeply I depended on my appearance to com-municate who I am to others, and resolved to reduce my reliance. And fourth, I recognized that, at least for me, looks-awareness—the watching, wanting, and wishing I was practicing in relation to beauty—is equivalent to lust.

Hungering after righteousness isn't automatic, I found: it's an acquired taste. And as long as I fed myself a continual diet of cheap substitutes, I never felt the gnaw-ing pangs of my conscience. It's only when I discovered that I'd been sold a false bill of goods—and *still* felt empty—that I cried out to God with my whole heart for His holy brand of satisfaction.

Now when I pray, "The Lord is my Shepherd; I shall not want," it isn't just about having a roof over my head or enough money to pay my bills or the next crisis looming on the horizon where I need God to meet me. It also applies to a need in my life I never once considered I should ask Jesus to fill: my inner secret longing for a real and lasting kind of beauty.

Turning Around

Breaking free from the beauty bind begins with over-coming this kind of denial. It isn't that caring about appearance is wrong—appearance is important and will continue to be. Instead, we need to understand why we've been seduced into serving beauty: we live in a world that promotes an obsessive preoccupation with appearance, especially the attractiveness of women.

Seeing the extent of our involvement is what can motivate us to want to change. "A person has to get fed up with the ways of the world before he, before she, acquires an appetite for the world of grace," says pastor Eugene Peterson in *A Long Obedience in the Same Direction.*[8] Of this, he writes:

> *Christian consciousness begins with the painful realization that what we had assumed was the truth is in fact a lie.* Prayer is immediate: "Deliver me, O LORD, from lying lips, from a deceitful tongue" (Psalm 120:1). Rescue me from the lies of advertisers who claim to know what I need and what I desire, from the lies of entertainers who promise a cheap way to joy. . . . The lies are impeccably factual. They contain no errors. There are no distortions or falsified data. But they are lies all the same because they claim to tell us who we are and omit everything about our origin in God and our destiny in God. They talk about the world without telling us that God made it. They tell us about our bodies without telling us that they are temples of the Holy Spirit. They instruct us in love without telling us about the God who loves us and gave himself for us.[9]

The usual biblical word describing the no we say to the world's lies and the yes we say to God's truth is repentance. . . . Repentance is not an emotion. It is not feeling sorry for your sins. It is deciding that you have been wrong in supposing that you could manage your own life and be your own god; it is deciding that you were wrong in thinking that you had, or could get, the strength, education and training to make it on your own; it is deciding that you have been told a pack of lies about yourself and your neighbor and your world. And it is deciding that God in Jesus Christ is telling you the truth. *Repentance is a realization that what God wants from you and what you want from God are not going to be achieved by doing the same*

*old things, thinking the same old thoughts. . . . It is a rejection that
is also an acceptance, a leaving that develops into an arriving, a
no to the world that is a yes to God.*[10]

Taking a reasonable amount of time to plan one's
wardrobe, create a pleasing appearance, or develop
sound dietary guidelines are all normal aspects of partici-
pating in our culture, as well as a way to enjoy and appreciate our God-given uniqueness. It's when our appearance and the appearance of others become a part of our
ongoing thoughts and feelings throughout the day, that
we jump from healthy self-care into looks-dependency.

Facing the extent of our participation with this way of
thinking and making the decision to change are the first
steps in the direction of repentance. Once we've done
this, we can begin finding the source of our femininity in
something bigger than how we look and what we wear.

From Dependence to Deliverance

Recently, while watching *Far and Away*, the story of Irish
immigrants coming to America in 1892, I was struck by the
washed-out look of many women appearing in the film. As
it turns out, in order to stay true to the time period, apparently none of the actresses playing Christian characters in
the movie could wear much makeup. (Only those in bur-
lesque dancers' roles wore heavily fortified eye-shadow
and lip color.) Even though I know women's use of cosmetics, expensive clothing, and jewelry isn't traditional
for church-going women, to my modern eyes these
Protestant ladies didn't look particularly feminine, they
looked *dowdy*. Without attractive clothes and cosmetics, I

wondered, how *do* women convey their femininity to those around them?

As I pondered this, I thought how often people today equate small sizes, clothing, cosmetics, and the appearance of youth with femininity. As an example, who would you choose as the more feminine woman: a petite, pretty 28-year-old woman with softly curled light brown hair wearing a size-four flowered sundress? Or a 65-year-old, 160 pound, gray-haired woman clothed in a loose-fitting cotton smock, thick elastic support hose, and heavy black shoes—with no makeup?

But what if the older woman happened to be Corrie Ten Boom and the younger one was Madonna? Who would you pick then as the more genuinely feminine woman of the two?

Femininity isn't what today's stereotypes suggest. To be feminine doesn't mean being a supple, attractively attired, vivacious ingenue—it's something far larger than this. At its highest and most noble, it is the reflective side of love. Femininity is also a fruit-bearing responsiveness to the Holy Spirit's infilling; wisdom working alongside will; intuition balancing action; creative skill infusing meaning into the mundane; the warmth of a nurturing embrace; a steadfast defense of the weak; and provision of shelter in the midst of a storm—the wings of a dove enfolding her young.[11]

Sexualized images of women fool us into thinking that womanliness has more to do with how we look than who we are. Consequently, it's much more challenging to be feminine without perfume, lipstick, or flowers than it is to depend on our appearance to express femininity to others.

The Colors of Virtue

In "The True Adornment of Women," St. John Chrysostom (c. 347-407) offers an unforgettable comparison of two opposing versions of feminine beauty: the outer "worldly" type versus inner spiritual beauty.

Reading these *Baptismal Instructions* for the first time, I reacted strongly to their seemingly "negative" tone toward women. But at the second reading, I saw something else entirely: the depth of my own reliance on clothing and cosmetics to make a favorable impression on others. By the time I'd read it again, I decided I really could wear less makeup to church, as well as elsewhere—and be better off for it. I've since gleaned a wealth of spiritual insight from thinking about these words, and pass them along to you for your own encouragement:

> Hereafter let there be no concern for external embellishments and expensive clothes, but let all your zeal be directed toward making your souls comely, that they may shine forth with a brighter beauty. Pay no attention to garments made from silkworm's threads, nor to necklaces of gold. For the teacher of the whole world, who knew full well the weakness of women's nature and the unsteadiness of their wills, did not hesitate to issue orders on these matters. Why do I say that he did not refuse to instruct you about these matters? While giving counsel to you women on your adornment, did he not cry out: *Not with braided hair or gold or pearls or expensive clothing?* Is not this all but an instruction concerning your desire to adorn yourselves and to win praise from those who behold you? I shall call not only on your fellow human beings but on the Master of all things to praise and honor you.[12]

We must, however, hear the exact words of the Apostle.

What, then, does he say? *But with good works such as become women professing godliness* (1 Timothy 2:10). Do deeds worthy of your profession, he says, and adorn yourself with good deeds. Let the good deeds you do imitate your profession; you profess godliness, so do what is pleasing to Him. What is this phrase "with good deeds"? He means the whole collection of virtues: scorn of this world, yearning for the world to come, disdain for riches, generosity to the poor, modesty, meekness, pursuit of wisdom, disposing our souls in peace and serenity, not cringing before the glory of the present life, but keeping our gaze ever straining upward, so that we are ever anxious for the things of heaven and desire the glory hereafter.[13]

Since I am now speaking especially to the women, I wish to make certain other recommendations to them. I wish you women to abstain not only from other hurtful practices, but also from the habit of painting your faces and adding to them, as if the workmanship were defective. By doing so, you insult the Workman. For what are you trying to do, woman? By using rouge and eye shadow you cannot add to your natural beauty nor change your natural ugliness, can you? These add nothing to your beauty of face, but they will destroy the beauty of your soul. For this meddling with nature testifies to your interior weakness. Especially are you heaping up abundant fire for yourself by exciting the looks of young men, and attracting to yourself the eyes of the undisciplined; by making complete adulterers of them, you are bringing their downfall on your head.[14]

It is fitting and helpful to abstain from this practice entirely. But if those women who are caught in the grip of this evil habit should be unwilling to give up the use of cosmetics, at least let them not use them when they are coming to the house of prayer. Why, tell me, when you come to church, do you adorn yourself in this way? You have come to worship God and to make confession to Him for atonement for your sins. Does He look for this beauty? No. He seeks the beauty from within, He looks for the activity which expresses itself in good deeds. He desires almsgiving, temperance, compunction, and strict faith.[15]

Do you wish to adorn your face? Do not do so with gems but with piety and modesty; thus adorned, a man will find your appearance more pleasing to behold. For that other adornment generally arouses suspicions which give rise to jealousy, enmity, strife, and quarrels. . . . Adorn your face, therefore with modesty, piety, almsgiving, benevolence, love, kindliness toward your husband, reasonableness, mildness, and forbearance. These are the pigments of virtue; by these, you draw not men but angels to you as your lovers; for these you have God Himself to praise you.[16]

But even if we should enjoy these things day in and day out, we shall be separated from them utterly by death. Virtue, however, does not change or alter; it is completely secure, and it both makes us more secure in this world and goes along with us to the next. Do you wish to possess pearls and never lay aside your wealth? Then strip off your adornment and put it into Christ's hands through the hands of His poor. Then He will put on you a better wealth and richer adornment, since your present wealth and adornment are really paltry and ridiculous.[17]

Think, then, who they are whom you wish to please and on whose account you wear this adornment. Is it that the ropemaker and the coppersmith and the man in the market may look at you and marvel? Are you not ashamed and do you not blush to be showing yourself off to these people and to be doing all this for men whom you do not consider worthy of a greeting?[18]

"The self is given to us that we may sacrifice it," George MacDonald once wrote. "It is ours, that we, like Christ, may have something to offer—not that we should torment it, but that we should deny it; not that we should cross it, but that we should abandon it utterly: then it can no more be vexed. . . . We are no more to think, 'What should I like to do?' but 'What would the Living One have me do?'"[19] It's easy to forget this question in a culture that substitutes sophistication for maturity, sleekness for femininity, and cardiovascular fitness for strength.

The Heart of the Matter

So, does this mean that after becoming believers we shouldn't wear any makeup at all? That we should adopt rigid dress codes, acquire trouser-free wardrobes, and abstain from wearing jewelry to avoid the "appearance of evil"? Or is it something more far-reaching—a moment-to-moment yielding of our hearts to God's rule as He changes our lives, from the inside out, to conform to His image within us?

The advice of St. John Chrysostom is valuable and contains timeless truths. But we also do well to remember that in our society, unlike in St. John's era, lipstick and mascara are worn by the majority of women—not just courtesans and prostitutes. Pants on women and gold earrings are acceptable to most Christians today, as is short hair. Resorting to stringent restrictions for the sake of promoting an appearance of femininity cheats us of our liberty in Christ, resulting in pride, judgmentalism, and hypocrisy—and can also prevent a deeper understanding of what real beauty is: the unfading loveliness of a calm and gentle spirit, a thing very precious in the eyes of God.[20]

"It is not enough that we inveigh against ourselves; we

must in a manner *forget* ourselves," wrote English evangelical Hannah More in an 1830 essay titled *Self-Love*.[21] To this, she adds:

> Christianity does not consist in an external conformity to practices which, though right in themselves, may be adopted from human motives and to answer secular purposes. It is not a religion of forms, modes, and decencies. It is being transformed into the image of God. It is being like-minded with Christ. It is considering Him as our sanctification as well as our redemption. It is endeavoring to live to Him here, that we may live with Him hereafter. It is desiring earnestly to surrender our will to His, our heart to the conduct of His Spirit, our life to the guidance of His Word.[22]

Christian discipleship offers us freedom and a fresh outlook as God invites us to simplify our lives and "worry not" about the hang-ups of our culture. In relationship to clothing and cosmetics, it means that we don't find our identity and worth in the things we wear, but in God. As John White explains:

> I believe that everything we do reflects our inner values and attitudes. Perhaps this should be our starting point. Too often, when we try to "dress Christian," we begin with dress and try to adjust our attitudes to fit our outward appearance, which is, of course, what man sees. And thus we elevate man's opinions above God's, who looks at our hearts . . .
>
> Whether women wear jewelry, make-up, have pierced ears or fake eyelashes, or whether men splash themselves with Musk, dangle gold chains around their necks, and wear Gucci shoes—these are not the basic issues. *What is significant is my peace of heart, my certainty that a loving God cares for me, and that dress is not the most important thing in the world.*[23]

We are not our own: we were bought with a price.[24]

Being "sold out" for Jesus doesn't come cheap: it's a costly, challenging, continual call to obedience and holiness. I've often heard it said that following Christ is like walking along a path or climbing up a mountain. But sometimes, it also means crossing swiftly running streams that threaten to knock us off our feet.

Yet in these troubled waters, *God provides us stepping stones.* In a balancing act of faith, He reaches His hand out toward us with the promise of never letting go, strengthening our ability to keep standing by His grace. As the rapid current of our culture dizzyingly dashes by, the sureness of His grip will remain steady and firm. Fixing our eyes on the truth of His Word, we can head forward with confidence in His direction—however faltering our steps may be—because we know that our Maker will not let us fall.

As women, whose ownership will we choose to reflect? How can our appearance be a witness to the Master we belong to? Since our hearts are found where our treasure lies, where are we most heavily invested? There are no fast or easy answers to these questions. Though Christ calls us to be childlike in our response to God's great love, He also reminds us that as His disciples we are to be "as shrewd as snakes and as innocent as doves."[25] In reading this book, I pray you've been greatly strengthened and encouraged to do both.

Remember: *You are most beautiful when you reflect the Lord's own beauty.* It's only in Jesus that we find out who we really are! Join me in rejoicing, won't you? And don't worry: the next time we meet, I won't be wondering about your weight.

❧ *Focus Questions* ❧

1. Why is simplicity a hallmark of the Christian life?
2. In what ways has reading this book encouraged you in your walk with God?
3. As you look forward to the future, what excites you most about where you're heading?

Epilogue

So, is it really possible to break free from beauty bondage? Now that you've nearly finished reading *Beauty and the Best*, it's a question worth asking.

Let me answer by encouraging you with the following story about a friend of mine. I first met Karen* about a dozen years ago after moving to Lincoln, Nebraska. She hadn't been a believer for very long—maybe two or three years. Yet one of the most remarkable things about her was that she already had a certain humility about her. Part of this, I suppose, was because of her understated clothing and pleasingly "ordinary" appearance. This isn't to say that Karen isn't beautiful. She is. But after becoming a Christian, she chose to no longer wear much make-up or spend a lot of money on her appearance. She prefers to stay busy investing her time and resources in God's Kingdom.

Looking at Karen, you would never guess that she had once been an active participant in today's beauty culture. It wasn't until I had known her for several years that she confided in me about her past. During her teens and 20s, Karen had lived with several men, had two abortions, and frequently used alcohol to numb her pain. She rarely talked about these experiences, but when she did, she always said something thought-provoking about the wonder of God's love and forgiveness at the same time.

In bits and pieces, I learned that Karen was well aware of the impact that her appearance can have on other people, but that she no longer wants to use her face and figure to attract or impress others. As a result, she is one of the few women I know who has made a conscious decision to deal with her tendencies toward vanity and covetousness regarding beauty.

There is a serenity about Karen that's comforting. When I'm with her, I'm not thinking about what she's wearing or how she looks—perhaps it's because she isn't thinking about it. Her well-groomed, relaxed appearance has a way of putting people at ease. Her clothes, while simple, are nicely designed and always appropriate for the occasion. Most importantly, by not drawing attention to her appearance, Karen's ministry to the Lord somehow shines more brightly. In her work within her church and community, she's a living example to me of what it means to be "transformed by grace."

You may know a few people like Karen. They're not the women who have never played the beauty game; they're just the ones who've quit. And they haven't dropped out because they don't care about the way they look—they do. But because they're intimately acquainted with the temptations of beauty, they know they can't follow Christ freely and still exalt false gods. They've let go of the fears that used to bind them and now laugh about their graying hair, dimpled thighs, chipped nails, stretch marks, and other insignificant physical imperfections.

Yes, it is possible to break free from the beauty bind, as Karen's life proves. But we need to want God's best for us, and that's sometimes the most difficult part of all. It's my hope that more women will find the courage to change, as Karen did, and present new images of beauty to the world, in all shapes, colors, and sizes.

* The name Karen is a pseudonym.

About the Author

Debra Evans writes, teaches, mothers her family, and watches football games with Dave, her husband of 23 years. Over the past two decades, more than 7,000 women have participated in Debra's classes, Bible studies, and weekend retreats.

A certified childbirth educator and contributing editor of *Christian Parenting Today* since 1988, she lives and works primarily at home in Austin, Texas, where three teenagers continually create interesting diversions that keep her days colorful.

A popular guest on Christian radio and television programs, Debra brings a refreshing blend of factual expertise and first-hand experience to her ministry, wherever she goes.

Beauty and the Best is Debra's tenth book.

ℬibliography

American Psychiatric Association. *Diagnostic and Statistical Manual of Mental Disorders.* 3rd ed., Washington, DC: 1980; 3rd ed., rev., Washington, DC, 1987.

Appleton, George. ed, *The Oxford Book of Prayer.* New York: Oxford University Press, 1985.

Atrens, Dale M. *Don't Diet.* New York: William Morrow, 1988.

Avon. *Looking Good, Feeling Beautiful: The Avon Book of Beauty.* New York: Simon and Schuster, 1981, p. 157.

Balsam, M. S. and Sagarin, Edward eds. *Cosmetic Science and Technology.* Vol. 3. New York: John Wiley, 1974.

Banner, Lois. *American Beauty.* New York: Alfred Knopf, 1983.

Begoun, Paula. *Blue Eyeshadow Should Be Illegal.* Seattle: Beginning Press, 1986.

·······················*Don't Go To The Cosmetics Counter Without Me.* Seattle: Beginning Press, 1991.

Bell, Rudolph M. *Holy Anorexia.* Chicago: University of Chicago, 1985.

Blumberg, Joan Jacobs. *Fasting Girls: The Emergence of Anorexia Nervosa as a Modern Disease.* Cambridge, MA: Harvard University Press, 1988.

Bowen-Woodward, Kathy. *Coping With a Negative Body-Image.* New York: Rosen Publishing Group, 1989.

Brand, Paul and Yancey, Philip. *In His Image.* Grand Rapids, MI: Zondervan, 1984.

Bray-Garretson, Helen and Cook, Kaye V. *Chaotic Eating: A Guide to Recovery.* Grand Rapids, MI: Zondervan, 1992.

Camp, John. *Plastic Surgery: The Kindest Cut.* New York: Henry Holt, 1989.

Caputi, Jane. *The Age of Sex Crime.* Bowling Green, OH: Bowling Green State University, Popular Press, 1987.

Chambers, Oswald. *My Utmost for His Highest.* New York: Dodd, Mead & Co., 1935.

Crichton, Michael. *Jurassic Park.* New York: Alfred Knopf, 1990.

Chrysostom, St. John. *Baptismal Instructions.* Westminster, MD: The Newman Press, 1963.

Colson, Charles. *Loving God.* Grand Rapids, MI: Zondervan, 1983.

Crewdson, John. *By Silence Betrayed: Sexual Abuse of Children.* New York: Harper & Row, 1988.

Dahl, Arlene. *Always Ask a Man: Arlene Dahl's Key to Femininity.* Englewood Cliffs, NJ: Prentice-Hall, 1965.

Evans, Debra. *Beauty for Ashes.* Wheaton, IL: Crossway Books, 1988.

···················· *Fragrant Offerings.* Wheaton, IL: Crossway Books, 1988.

···················· *The Mystery of Womanhood.* Wheaton, IL: Crossway Books, 1987.

Freedman, Rita. *Age Before Beauty.* New York: Peter Pauper Press, 1991.

···················· *Beauty Bound.* Lexington, MA: Lexington Books, 1986.

Graham, J. A. and Kligman, A. M. eds. *The Psychology of Cosmetic Treatments.* New York: Prager Scientific, 1985.

Hatfield, E. and Sprecher, Susan, *Mirror. Mirror . . . The Importance of Looks in Everyday Life.* Albany, NY: State Unversity of New York Press, 1986.

Hunt, Gladys. *Ms. Means Myself.* Grand Rapids, MI: Zondervan, 1972.

Hutton, Deborah. *Vogue Complete Beauty.* London: Octupus Books, 1982.

Keyes, Dick. *Beyond Identity.* Ann Arbor, MI: Servant Books, 1984.

❧ Bibliography ❧

Lakoff, Robin Tomlach and Scherr, Roberta L. *Face Value: The Politics of Beauty.* Boston: Routledge and Kegan Paul, 1984.

Lewis, C. S. *George MacDonald: An Anthology.* New York: Macmillan, 1947.

.... *That Hideous Strength.* New York: Macmillan, 1965.

.... "The Weight of Glory," in *The Weight of Glory.* Grand Rapids, MI: Eerdmans, 1975.

Liggett, John. *The Human Face.* New York: Stein and Day, 1974.

Marwick, Arthur. *Beauty in History.* New York: Thames & Hudson, 1988.

McGee, Robert. *The Search for Significance.* Houston: Rapha, 1990.

Morgan, Elizabeth. *The Complete Book of Cosmetic Surgery.* New York: Warner, 1988.

Morton, Andrew. *Diana's Diary: An Intimate Portrait of the Princess of Wales.* New York: Summit Books, 1990.,

Overduin, Daniel and Fleming, John. *Life in a Test-Tube.* Adelaide, South Australia: Lutheran Publishing House, 1982.

Patzer, G. L. *The Physical Attractiveness Phenomena.* New York: Plenum Press, 1985.

Peterson, Eugene H. *A Long Obedience in the Same Direction: Discipleship in an Instant Society.* Downer's Grove, IL: InterVarsity Press, 1980.

Piper, John. *Desiring God.* Portland, OR: Multnomah Press, 1986.

Plato. *The Collected Dialogues.* Edith Hamilton and Huntington Cairns, eds. Princeton, NJ: Princeton University Press, 1963.

Plaut, W. Gunther, ed. *The Torah: A Modern Commentary.* New York: Union of American Hebrew Congregations, 1981.

Random House College Dictionary. rev. ed. New York: Random House, 1984.

Rodin, Judith. *Body Traps: Breaking the Binds That Keep You From Feeling Good About Your Body.* New York: William Morrow, 1992.

Rodin, Judith, Silberstein, Lisa, and Striegel-Moore, Ruth. "Women and Weight: A Normative Discontent," in *1984 Nebraska*

Symposium on Motivation. ed. Theodore B. Sondregger Lincoln, 1985.

Secunda, Victoria. *By Youth Possessed: The Denial of Age in America.* Indianapolis: Bobbs-Merrill, 1984.

Seid, Roberta Pollack. *Never Too Thin: Why Women Are at War with Their Bodies.* New York: Prentice Hall, 1989.

Schwartz, Hillel. *Never Satisfied: A Cultural History of Diets, Fantasies, and Fat.* New York: The Free Press/Macmillan, 1986.

Solomon, M., ed. *The Psychology of Fashion.* Lexington, MA: Lexington Books, 1985.

Sproul, R. C. *Pleasing God.* Wheaton, IL: Tyndale, 1988.

Standard and Poor's Industry Surveys. New York: Standard and Poor's Corp., 1988.

Steer, Roger ed. *The George Müeller Treasury.* Wheaton, IL: Crossway Books, 1987.

Stott, John R. W. *Christian Counter-Culture: The Message of the Sermon on the Mount.* Downer's Grove, IL: InterVarsity Press, 1978.

Taylor, Debbie, et al. *Women: A World Report.* Oxford: Oxford University Press, 1985.

White, John., *Changing on the Inside.* Ann Arbor, MI: Vine Books, 1991.

······················ *Flirting with the World.* Downer's Grove, IL: InterVarsity Press, 1982.

······················ *The Fight.* Downer's Grove, IL: InterVarsity Press, 1978.

Wirt, Sherwood Eliot. *Spiritual Awakening.* Wheaton, IL: Crossway Books, 1986.

Wolf, Naomi. *The Beauty Myth.* New York: William Morrow, 1991.

Endnotes

Research for Beauty and the Best *included the extensive use of popular and academic sources, in addition to scriptural study. My use of secular references, however, is not meant to imply my endorsement of any book, journal, televison network, newspaper, or magazine cited below.*

Chapter 1

- Arthur Marwick, *Beauty in History* (New York: Thames and Hudson, 1988), 37.

1. K. W. Woods, "Cindy Crawford: I'm Afraid Men Will Leave Me," *Woman's World,* 6 Aprl. 1993, 39.

2. Elizabeth Sporkin, "The Body Game," *People Weekly,* 11 Jan. 1993, 80-86.

3. Sporkin, "The Body Game," 81.

4. Sporkin, "The Body Game," 82 and 83.

5. Sporkin, "The Body Game." 82.

6. Sporkin, "The Body Game," 82 and 84.

7. Sporkin, "The Body Game," 83.

8. Sporkin, "The Body Game," 81 and 84.

9. E. Walster et al., "Importance of Physical Attractiveness in Dating Behavior," *Journal of Personality and Social Psychology* 4 (1966): 508-516; W. J. Dibiase and L. A. Hjelle, "Body-Image Stereotypes and Body-Type Preferences Among Male College Students,"

Perceptual and Motor Skills 27 (1968): 1143-1146; A. G. Miller, "Role of Physical Attractiveness in Impression Formation," *Psychonomic Science* 19 (1970): 241-243; E. Berscheid, K. K. Dion, E. Walster, and G. W. Walster, "Physical Attractiveness and Dating Choice," *Journal of Experimental Social Psychology* 7 (1971): 173-189; E. Berscheid et al., "What Is Beautiful Is Good," *Journal of Personality and Social Psychology* 24 (1972): 285-290; H. Sigall and E. Aronson, "Radiating Beauty: The Effects of Having a Physically Attractive Partner on Person Perception," *Journal of Personality and Social Psychology* 28 (1973): 218-224; D. Landy and H. Sigall, "Beauty Is Talent: Task Evaluation as a Function of the Performer's Physical Attractiveness," *Journal of Personality and Social Psychology* 29 (1974): 299-304; K. K. Dion, "The Incentive Value of Physical Attractiveness," *Personality and Social Psychology Bulletin* 3 (1977): 67-70; G. R. Adams and S. M. Crossman, *Physical Attractiveness: A Cultural Imperative* (Roslyn Heights, NY: Libra, 1978); K. K. Dion, "Physical Attractiveness, Sex Roles and Heterosexual Attraction," in M. Cook, ed., *The Bases of Human Sexual Attraction* (London: Academic Press, 1981), 3-22; T. F. Cash and L. H. Janda, "The Eye of the Beholder," *Psychology Today*, Dec. 1984, 46-52; M. L. Barnes and R. Rosenthal, "Interpersonal Effects of Eexperimenter Attractiveness, Attire, and Gender," *Journal of Personality and Social Psychology* 48 (1985): 435-46; E. Hatfield and S. Sprecher, *Mirror, Mirror . . . the Importance of Looks in Everyday Life* (Albany, NY: State University of New York Press, 1986); S. Sprecher, "The Importance to Males and Females of Physical Attractiveness, Earning Potential, and Expressiveness in Initial Attraction," *Sex Roles: A Journal of Research* 21 (1989): 591-608; J. Camp, "The Importance of Being Pretty," *Health*, June 1989, 80-84; A. C. Downs, "Objective and Subjective Physical Attractiveness Judgements among Young Adults," *Perceptual and Motor Skills* (70) 1990: 458; C. R. Jasper and M. L. Klassen, "Perceptions of Salespersons' Appearance and Evaluation of Job Performance," *Perceptual and Motor Skills* 71 (1990): 563-566; C. R. Jasper and M. L. Klassen, "Stereotypical Beliefs about Appearance: Implications for Retailing and Consumer Issues," *Perceptual and Motor Skills* 71 (1990): 519-528; A.

H. Eagly et al., and L. Longo, "What Is Beautiful Is Good, But . . . : A Meta-analytic Review of Research on the Physical Attractiveness Stereotype," *Psychology Bulletin* 110 (1991), 109-129; S. Garcia et al., "Shyness and Physical Attractiveness in Mixed-Sex Dyads," *Journal of Personality and Social Psychology* 61 (1991), 35-50; M. D. Gynther, A. T. Davis, and L. G. Shake, "The Perception of Attractiveness: What About the Beholders?" *Journal of Clinical Psychology* 47 (1991): 745-749.

10. Quoted by Rita Freedman, *Age Before Beauty* (New York: Peter Pauper Press, Inc.,1991): 56.

11. Romans 7:15,18.

12. Freedman, *Beauty Bound,* 7.

13. See 1 Corinthians 10:13, for example.

14. Romans 12:1-2; 1 John 1:16; Ephesians 6:12; 2 Timothy 3:1-5.

15. Romans 8:1.

16. Genesis 12:10 through13:2; 20:1 thru 21:7; Genesis 29:1-30; 2 Samuel 11:1 thru 12:25; the book of Esther.

17. 1 Thessalonians 5:24.

18. Reported by Jill Rappaport on NBC News, *Today,* 17 Feb.1993; *The Atlanta Journal,* "Swimsuit Issue Out Today," 17 Feb. 1993.

19. Each month, women's magazines are heavy on female nudity, pictured in alluring layouts promoting everything from the latest skin care treatments to Calvin Klein underwear. Advertisements for perfume and cosmetics regularly feature models' faces that suggestively imply sexual delight. As a result, the similarity between women modeling as a sales pitch to women and women posing to attract male magazine buyers seems to have never been blurrier—or stronger.

   In a recent article, *USA Today* articulately points out that the careers of models such as Cindy Crawford, Joan Severance, and Stephanie Seymour received a big boost via *Playboy* pictorials [Ann Trebbe, "Timing Is All When Baring for '*Playboy*,'" 26 Apr.

1993, 1D], an interesting twist to the erotic emphasis of today's image cult. Beyond this, let's not forget: pornography generates an estimated 7 billion dollars worldwide every year—more than all the revenues brought in from the legitimate film and music industries combined.

In the past 15 years, this industry has increased 1,600 times over and now has more "franchises" than McDonald's. So-called "porn flicks" now outnumber other films by three to one, and gross one million dollars a day in the United States alone.

See: J. Galloway and J. Thornton, "Crackdown on Pornography—A No-Win Battle," *U.S. News & World Report*, 4 June 1984, 84-85; T. Minnery, "Pornography: The Human Tragedy," *Christianity Today*, March 7, 1986, 17-22; T. Minnery, "What It Takes to Fight Pornography," *Christianity Today*, February 15, 1985, 10-11; A. Press et al., "The War Against Pornography," *Newsweek*, 18 Mar. 1985, 58-67; J. Caputi, *The Age of Sex Crime* (Bowling Green, OH: Bowling Green State University, Popular Press, 1987); D. Taylor et al., *Women: A World Report* (Oxford: Oxford University Press, 1985), 67; J. B. Weaver, J. L. Masland, and D. Zillmann, "Effect of Erotica on Young Men's Aesthetic Perception of Their Female Sexual Partners," *Perceptual and Motor Skills* 58 (1984): 929-930; D. T. Kenrick and S. E. Gutierres, "Influence of Popular Erotica on Judgments of Strangers and Mates," *Journal of Experimental Social Psychology* 25 (1989): 159-168; V. R. Padgett, J. A. Brislin-Slutz, and J. A. Neal, "Pornography, Erotica, and Attitudes Toward Women: The Effects of Repeated Exposure," *The Journal of Sex Research* 26 (1989): 479-492; D. F. Duncan, "Violence and Degradation as Themes in 'Adult' Videos," *Psychological Reports* 69 (1991): 239-241; J. Norris, "Social Influence Effects on Responses to Sexually Explicit Material Containing Violence," *The Journal of Sex Research* 28 (1991), 67-77; R. W. Bennett and D. F. Gates, "The Relationship Between Pornography and Extrafamilial Child Sexual Abuse," *The Police Chief* 58 (1991):14-18.

Chapter 2

- Tamara Eberlein, "Learning to Love Your Body," *First for Women*, 15 Mar.1993, 38.

1. Judith Newman, "Straight from the Hip: The Truth About Liposuction," *Mirabella*, July 1992, 64.

2. Marwick, *Beauty in History*, 17.

3. Marwick, *Beauty in History*, 13.

4. *Standard and Poor's Industry Surveys* (New York: Standard and Poor's Corp., 1988); Molly O'Neill, "Congress Looking into Diet Business," *The New York Times*, 28 Mar.1990; David Brand, "A Nation of Healthy Worrywarts?" Time, 25 July 1988; Freedman, *Beauty Bound*, 43.

5. Marwick, *Beauty in History*, 60-61.

6. Mark Muro, "A New Era of Eros in Advertising," *The Boston Globe*, 16 Apr. 1986. These commercials, in turn, directly influence women's views of their own bodies. See: P. N. Myers and F. A. Biocca, "The Elastic Body Image: The Effect of Television Advertising and Programming on Body Image Distortions in Young Women," *Journal of Communication* 42 (1992): 108-132; and K. L. Nagel and K. H. Jones, "Sociological Factors in the Development of Eating Disorders," *Adolescence* 27 (1992): 107-114.

7. Magazine Publishers of America, "Magazine Advertising Revenue by Class Totals, Jan. Dec. 1989," Information Bureau, A. H. B., Jan. 1990.

8. John Crewdson, *By Silence Betrayed: Sexual Abuse of Children* (New York: Harper & Row, 1988), 249.

9. David Garner et al., "Cultural Expectation of Thinness in Women," *Psychological Reports*, 47 (1980): 483-491.

10. Roberta Pollack Seid, *Never Too Thin: Why Women Are at War with Their Bodies* (New York: Prentice Hall, 1989), 15.

11. Paula England, Alice Kuhn, and Teresa Gardner, "The Ages of Men and Women in Magazine Advertisements," *Journalism Quarterly*, Autumn 1981, 468-471.

12. Susan Jacoby, "The Body Image Blues," *Family Circle*, 1 Feb. 1990, 41-46.

13. Jacoby, "The Body Image Blues," 41-46.

14. Jacoby, "The Body Image Blues," 42.

15. Irene Daria, "Truth in Fashion," *Glamour*, Feb. 1993, 149.

    It is important to remember that in the late 1800's, the American beauty ideal was represented by a woman with a 36-26-38 figure—a far cry from Twiggy's 92-pound frame.

16. Pollack Seid, *Never Too Thin*, 3-4.

17. A. T. Fleming, "Living Dolls," *Allure*, Mar.1991, 132.

18. Elaine L. Pedersen and Nancy L. Markee, "Fashion Dolls: Representations of Ideals of Beauty," *Perceptual and Motor Skills* 73 (1991): 93-94.

19. Laura Shapiro, "What Is It with Women and Breasts?" *Newsweek*, 20 Jan. 1992, 57.

20. Naomi Wolf, *The Beauty Myth* (New York: William Morrow and Company, Inc. 1991), 59.

Chapter 3

- Madame Bayard, quoted in Marwick, *Beauty in History*, 230.

- Lois Wyse, "The Way We Are," *Good Housekeeping*, June 1991, 226.

1. These calculations were based on a 10-hour retailing day, 365 days per year, by Kline and Co. Quoted in "What Price Beauty?" *Glamour*, Apr. 1991, 297.

2. Marshall L. Raines, "Status and Structure of the Cosmetics Industry," in M. S. Balsam and Edward Sagarin, eds., *Cosmetic Science and Technology*, vol. 3 (New York: John Wiley, 1974) and *Standard and Poor's Industry Surveys*, H34-35.

3. Paula Begoun, *Blue Eyeshadow Should Be Illegal* (Seattle: Beginning Press, 1986), 13.

4. "Shampoos & Conditioners," *Consumer Reports*, Jun. 1992, 395.

After testing shampoos and conditioners on nearly 20 pounds of human hair, tied into more than 1,000 ponytails, *CR* rated 132 different brands of shampoos and conditioners. Topping the list—surprise, surprise!—were inexpensive mass-marketed products such as White Rain Extra Body, White Rain Plus, Suave Shampoo Plus Conditioner, Rave All In One, Pert Plus, Alberto VO5 Conditioner for Permed/Color-Treated Hair, and Faberge Organics, along with the more expensive salon-marketed Paul Mitchell Shampoo Three and Nexxus Ensure.

5. Begoun, *Blue Eyeshadow*, 14.

6. Pat Sloan, "Mass-Market Clarion to get Image Boost," *Advertising Age*, 6 Jan. 1992, 3.

7. Ingredients in cosmetics must be listed clearly on all product packaging, making it easier for consumers to compare products and avoid allergens, such as urea, lanolin, and PABA—that is, *if* one knows what to look for. The ingredients that are most beneficial for dry skin, grouped by chemical similarities, are: *allantonin* (heals and soothes skin); *amino acids* and *proteins* (makes skin smoother); *animal collagen* and *animal elastin* (keeps water in skin); *cholesterol, fatty acids* such as stearic acid, tea-stearate, glyceryl stearate SE, *lecithin, phospholipids,* and *triglycerides* (binds water to skin); *glycerin* (attracts water to skin); *glycosamino-glycans, hyaluronic acid,* and *mucopolysaccharides* (helps water penetrate skin); *lanolin* (keeps skin soft and supple, but avoid it if you're allergic to wool); *liposomes* (retains water and skin's natural oils); *mineral oil* and *petrolatum* (holds water in skin; this group also includes *apricot kernel, avocado, basil, carrot, castor, coconut, egg, geranium, jojoba, lanolin, lavender, macadamia, olive, palm, peppermint, rice bran, safflower, sandalwood, sesame, shark, soybean, sunflower, and sweet almond oils); propylene glycol, butylene glycol and polyethylene glycol* or *PEG* (attracts moisture and helps cream spread over skin); *sodium pca* (holds water in skin); *tocopherol* or *vitamin E* (an antioxidant that repels oxygen and prevents skin dehydration), and *water* (the most important skin nutrient of all). The following ingredients boost product prices substantially, but have *no proven ability* to help skin hold moisture and have not been shown in

independent research to benefit skin: *amniotic fluid; plant, marine or animal extracts; placental protein;* and *serums.*

8. Paula Begoun, "Don't Go to the Cosmetic Counter Without Me," (Seattle: Beginning Press, 1991).

9. Victoria Geibel, "Vogue Beauty: Mascara, Never More Popular," *Vogue,* Aug. 1991, 190.

10. Gretchen Morgenson, "How Different Can a $17 Lipstick Be From a $3 Version?" *Forbes,* 18 Sept. 1989, 129.

11. Morgenson, "How Different Can a $17 Lipstick Be?" 129.

12. Pat Sloan, "Blond Faith in the '90s," *Advertising Age,* 6 Jan. 1992, 3.

13. Sloan, "Blond Faith in the '90s," 3.

14. "What Price Beauty?" 296.

15. "What Price Beauty?" 296.

16. "What Price Beauty?" 302.

17. Avon, *Looking Good, Feeling Beautiful: The Avon Book of Beauty* (New York: Simon and Schuster, 1981), 157.

18. Deborah Hutton, *Vogue Complete Beauty* (London: Octopus Books, 1982), 11.

19. Anthony Synnott, "Truth and Goodness, Mirrors and Masks—Part I: A Sociology of Beauty and the Face," *The British Journal of Sociology* 40 (1989): 607. [For additional commentary and research on the use of cosmetics, see also: E. T. Wright et al., "Some Psychological Effects of Cosmetics," *Perceptual and Motor Skills* (30) 1970: 12-14; L. Theberge and A. Kernaleguen, "Importance of Cosmetics Related to Aspects of the Self," *Perceptual and Motor Skills* (48) 1979: 827-830; J. A. Graham and A. J. Jouhar, "The Effects of Cosmetics on Personal Perception," *International Journal of Cosmetics Science* (2) 1981: 199-210; T. F. Cash and D. W. Cash, "Women's Use of Cosmetics: Psychological Correlates and Consequences," *International Journal of Cosmetic Science* (4) 1982: 1-14; J. A. Graham and A. M. Kligman, eds., *The Psychology of Cosmetic Treatments* (New York: Prager Scientific, 1985); T. F. Cash, J. Rissi, and R. Chapman, "Not Just Another

Pretty Face: Sex Roles, Locus of Control, and Cosmetics Use," *Personality and Social Psychology Bulletin* (9) 1985; 246-257; T. F. Cash: "The Psychology of Cosmetics: A Review of the Scientific Literature," *Social and Behavioral Sciences Documents* (17) 1987; 1. (Ms. No. 2800); T. F. Cash, "The Psychology of Cosmetics: A Research Bibliography," *Perceptual and Motor Skills* (66) 1988; 455-460; T. F. Cash et al., "Effects of Cosmetics on the Physical Attractiveness and Body Image of American College Women," *Journal of Social Psychology* (129) 1988: 349-355.

Chapter 4

- Kathy Bowen-Woodward, *Coping With a Negative Body-Image* (New York: Rosen Publishing Group, 1989).

1. Pollack Seid, *Never Too Thin*, 3.

2. Pollack Seid, *Never Too Thin*, 4.

3. Pollack Seid, *Never Too Thin*, 3-4.

4. Jeffrey Zaslow, "Fourth-Grade Girls These Days Ponder Weighty Matters," *The Wall Street Journal*, 11 Feb. 1986, 1, 20; *The Chronicle of Higher Education*, 19 Nov. 1986, 11-12; and Michael Prestage, "Narrow Minded," *Times Educational Supplement*, 20 Sept. 1991, 27. Fat-phobic attitudes among young children shouldn't surprise adults. In a special issue on the American family published in Winter 1990, *Newsweek* magazine reported on a study of 200 couples conducted by the New England Genetics Research Group: whereas two of the couples responding said they would have an abortion on the basis of sex alone—and 12 claimed they would abort a child who was likely to develop Alzheimer's disease—22 said they would terminate their child's life due to his or her genetic predisposition to obesity.

For more information concerning the scope of fat-hating in America, see: Gina Kolata, "The Burdens of Being Overweight," *The New York Times*, 22 Nov. 1992, N1 and L1; Daniel Seligman, "Fat chances," *Fortune*, 20 May 1991, 155-157; D. M. Czajka-Narins and E. S. Parham, "Fear of Fat: Attitudes Toward Obesity,"

Nutrition Today, 25 (1990), 26-33; and C. Crandall and M. Biernat, "The Ideology of Anti-Fat Attitudes," *Journal of Applied Social Psychology*, 20 (1990): 227-240.

5. Linda J. Murray, "Nutrition News: The High Cost of Losing Weight," *First for Women*, 5 Apr. 1993, 22. Other eating disorder-related symptoms include: *irregular menstruation; unexplained disappearance of household food (especially sweets); deepening preoccupation with physical appearance, accompanied by comments like, "I hate my body," and "I'm so fat"; regularly showering after meals (masks vomiting); compulsive preoccupation with exercise; and sudden interest and fascination with dieting books and cookbooks.* If you suspect that your child or someone you know has an eating disorder, consult a doctor or therapist for advice on how to help. See also: Dixie Farley, "Eating Disorders Require Medical Attention," *FDA Consumer*, Mar. 1992, 27-30; K. L. Nagel and K. H. Jones, "Predisposition Factors in Anorexia Nervosa," *Adolescence* 27 (1992): 381-387; K. A. Halmi, J. E. Mitchell, and N. A. Rigotti, "Anorexia and Bulimia: You Can Help," *Patient Care*, Mar. 30, 1993, 24-39; M. Grodner, "'Forever Dieting': Chronic Dieting Syndrome," *Journal of Nutrition Education* 24 (1992): 204-211; R. L. Horne, J. C. Van Vactor, and S. Emerson, "Disturbed Body Image in Patients with Eating Disorders," *American Journal of Psychiatry* 148 (1991): 210-215; and J. T. Kerr, R. L. Skok, and T. F. McLaughlin, "Characteristics Common to Females Who Exhibit Anorexic or Bulimic Behavior: A Review of the Current Literature," *Journal of Clinical Psychology* 47 (1991): 846-854.

6. American Psychiatric Association, *Diagnostic and Statistical Manual of Mental Disorders* 3rd ed. (Washington, D.C.,1980): 3rd ed., rev. (Washington, D.C., 1987).

7. Katherine A. Halmi, "Anorexia Nervosa: Recent Investigations," *Annual Review of Medicine* 29 (1978): 20,137-148; C. G. Banks, "'Culture' in Culture-Bound Syndromes: The Case of Anorexia Nervosa," *Social Science & Medicine* 34 (1992): 867-885; M. J. Cooper and C. G. Fairburn, "Thoughts About Eating, Weight, and Shape in Anorexia Nervosa and Bulimia Nervosa," *Behavior Research and Therapy* 30 (1992): 501-512; Don Dunn, "When Thinness Becomes

Illness," *Business Week* 3 Aug.1992, 74-76; D. L. Tobin et. al., "Multifactorial Assessment of Bulimia Nervosa," *Journal of Abnormal Psychology* 100 (1991): 14-22; and Joan Jacobs Blumberg, *Fasting Girls: The Emergence of Anorexia Nervosa as a Modern Disease* (Cambridge, MA: Harvard University Press, 1988), 258.

AA/BA materials also state that anorexia nervosa and bulimia strike more than 1,000,000 American women annually. During the 1980s, there were 17,024 more deaths from anorexia than from AIDS (until the end of 1988). But who would know that more than one million women have died of anorexia in the past decade? The ravages AIDS wreaks on the human body are broadcast regularly as the media promotes "safe" sex to save lives. Yet, at the same time, it continues to feed women a steady visual diet of emaciated beauty images to emulate, thereby directly contributing to the anorexia-related death toll. Why aren't more women outraged by this?

8. For an in-depth account of anorexia in medieval women, read Rudolph M. Bell, *Holy Anorexia* (Chicago: University of Chicago, 1985). Bell, a professor of history at Rutgers Univeristy, contends that three distinct types of anorexia prevailed among Christian "holy women" between 1200 and 1500, the most extreme of which led to death by self-starvation and "related harsh austerities."

9. Bell, *Holy Anorexia,* 22-83. See also: A. Stunkard, "A Description of Eating Disorders in 1932," *American Journal of Psychiatry* 147 (1990): 263-269; and B. Thornton, R. Leo, and K. Alberg, "Gender Role Typing, the Superwoman Ideal, and the Potential for Eating Disorders," *Sex Roles: A Journal of Research* 25 (1991): 469-485.

10. Caroline Walker Bynum, *Holy Feast and Holy Fast: Food Motifs in the Piety of Medieval Women,* cited in Blumberg, 45; see also: Caroline Walker Bynum, "Fast, Feast, and Flesh: The Religious Significance of Food to Medieval Women," *Representations* 11 (1985): 1-25.

11. Bell, *Holy Anorexia, x.*

12. See Ecclesiastes 3:13, for example.

13. Romans 14:15; see also Matthew 6:25-34; 1 Corinthians 10:31.

14. Dale M. Artens, *Don't Diet* (New York: William Morrow and Company, Inc., 1988): 15-16. See also: "Losing Weight: What Works, What Doesn't," *Consumer Reports,* June 1993, 347-352; Frederick K. Goodwin, "Need to Lose Weight? Oh Rats!" *JAMA, The Journal of the American Medical Association* 267 (1992): 910; Ruth Papazian, "Never Say Diet?" *FDA Consumer,* Oct. 1991, 8; C. Bouchard et. al., "The Response to Long-Term Overfeeding in Identical Twins," *The New England Journal of Medicine* 322 (1990): 1477-1483; A. J. Stunkard et al., "The Body-Mass Index of Twins Who Have Been Reared Apart," *The New England Journal of Medicine* 322 (1990): 1483-1488; Editorial, "Destiny Rides Again as Twins Overeat: Inheritance of Obesity Studies in Twins," *The New England Journal of Medicine* 322 (1990): 1522-1525; "Born To Be Fat?" *U. S. News & World Report,* 14 May 1990, 62; S. C. Wooley and D. M. Garner, "Obesity Treatment: The High Cost of False Hope," *Journal of the American Dietetic Association* 91 (1991): 1248-1252; and Gina Kolata, "Where Fat Is the Problem, Heredity Is the Answer, Studies Find," *The New York Times,* 24 May 1990.

15. Lori Miller Kase, "Weight Game," *Bazaar,* Apr. 1993, 291.

16. Nanci Hellmich, "Innovative Fat-Fighter Jean Nidetch," *USA Today,* 18 May 1993, 1D.

17. Hellmich, "Innovative Fat-Fighter," 2D. According to *USA Today,* commercial weight-loss programs represented a $2 billion-per-year industry in 1990; projected growth of sales for 1996 is estimated at $3.2 billion dollars. Based on an average 24 pound loss, a recent survey revealed what it costs when the following programs and procedures are used. (Figures in parentheses represent weekly food costs.) Liposuction: $2,000-$4,000; one week at Canyon Ranch Spa in Arizona, including food: $3,908; Nutri-System: $980 ($72); Jenny Craig: $840 ($66); Weight Watchers: $786 ($40-$60); your own plan $500 ($40-$60); one black figure-flattering dress: $59. [Source: Murray, op. cit. See also: "Rating the Diets," *Consumer Reports,* June 1993, 353-357.]

18. Laura Fraser, "The Death of Dieting," *Vogue*, May 1993, 293.

19. "Rating the Diets," *Consumer Reports*, 357.

20. "Rating the Diets," *Consumer Reports*, 357.

21. Hillel Schwartz, *Never Satisfied: A Cultural History of Diets, Fantasies, and Fat* (New York: The Free Press/Macmillan, 1986), 321-322. See also: Jane E. Brody, "For Most Trying to Lose Weight, Dieting Only Makes Things Worse," *The New York Times*, 23 Nov. 1992, A1; Janet Raloff, "Cyclic Weight Gain May Harm the Heart," *Science News*, 29 June 1991, 407; C. D. Berdanier and M. K. McIntosh, "Weight Loss—Weight Regain: A Vicious Cycle," *Nutrition Today* 26 (1991): 6-13; "Long-Term Problems with Weight-Loss Programs," *Consumer's Research Magazine*, July 1992, 22-26.

22. Orlando Wayne Wooley and Susan C. Wooley, "33,000 Women Tell Us How They Really Feel About Their Bodies," *Glamour*, Feb.1984. See also: Susan C. Wooley and Orlando Wayne Wooley, "Obesity and Women I: A Closer Look at the Facts," *Women's Studies International Quarterly* 2 (1979): 69-79.

23. Bowen-Woodward, *Coping with a Negative Body-Image*, 7-8.

24. Assessment based on Bowen-Woodward, *Coping with a Negative Body Image*, 10-11.

25. For further information, I suggest you read: Helen Bray-Garretson and Kaye V. Cook, *Chaotic Eating: A Guide to Recovery* (Grand Rapids, MI: Zondervan, 1992); Jane R. Hirschmann and Carol H. Hunter, *Overcoming Overeating* (New York: Fawcett Columbine/Ballantine Books, 1988); Frank Minirth et al., *Love Hunger* (Nashville, TN: Thomas Nelson Publishers, 1990); and Jan Johnson, *When Food Is Your Best Friend (& Worst Enemy)* (San Francisco: HarperCollins Publishers, 1993).

26. Fraser, "The Death of Dieting," 292.

27. Marjorie Rosen et al., "Big Gain, No Pain," *People Weekly*, 14 Jan. 1991, 82, 85.

28. Marjorie Rosen, "For Delta, Roseanne and TV's Other Big Talents, Heavy Means High Ratings," *People Weekly*, 14 Jan. 1991, 88.

29. Frank Sanello, "In the Hot Seat: Delta Burke," *Woman's World,* 1 June 1993, 18.

30. Elizabeth Sporkin, "A Terrible Hunger," *People Weekly,* 17 Feb. 1992, 94.

31. Sporkin, "A Terrible Hunger," 95.

32. See Romans 12:2.

33. Philippians 3:12.

34. Fraser, "The Death of Dieting," 330.

35. Fraser, "The Death of Dieting," 347-352; Debra Waterhouse, "Outsmarting the Female Fat Cell," *Good Housekeeping,* May 1993, 60, 73-75; Leslie Laurence, "How Oprah (and You) Can Lose Weight for Good," *McCall's,* Jan. 1992, 14-16; "Body Fat: The Hormone Factor," *Science News,* 15 June 1991, 383; Jules Hirsch, "The Puzzle of Fat Cells," *Healthline,* Dec.1991, 213-216; Gordon Bakoulis Bloch, "The Victorious Dieter: To Win the Battle of the Bulge, You Must Overcome the Forces of Nature," *Health,* Oct. 1990, 36-39; and Gina Kolata, "One Reason Why it's Hard to Keep Off Lost Weight," *The New York Times,* 12 Apr. 1990, B7. See also: P. A. Kern et al., "The Effects of Weight Loss on Activity and Expression of Adipose-Tissue Lipoprotein Lipase in Very Obese Humans," *The New England Journal of Medicine* 322 (1990): 1053-1063; M. U. Yang, E. Presta, and P. Bjorntorp, "Refeeding after Fasting in Rats: Effects of Duration of Starvation and Refeeding on Food Efficiency in Diet-Induced Obesity," *American Journal of Clinical Nutrition* 51 (1990): 970-979; and A. G. Duloo and L. Girardier, "Adaptive Changes in Energy Expenditure During Refeeding Following Low-Calorie Intake: Evidence for a Specific Metabolic Component Favoring Fat Storage," *American Journal of Clinical Nutrition* 52 (1990): 415-422.

36. Fraser, "The Death of Dieting," 330.

37. D. J. A. Jenkins et al., "Nibbling Versus Gorging: Metabolic Advantages of Increased Meal Frequency," *The New England Journal of Medicine* 321 (1989): 929-934.

Chapter 5

- Marjorie Rosen et al., "On the Cutting Edge," *People Weekly*, 27 Jan. 1992, 63.

1. Wolf, *The Beauty Myth*, 231-232.

2. M. Edgerton, M. Jacobson, and E. Meyer, "Surgical-Psychiatric Study of Patients Seeking Plastic Surgery," *British Journal of Plastic Surgery* 13 (1961): 136-145.

3. Statistics in this paragraph may be found in: *Standard and Poor's Industry Surveys*, Steven Findlay, "Buying the Perfect Body," *U.S. News & World Report*, 1 May 1989, 68; Susan Jacoby, "Appearance Anxiety," *The New York Times Magazine*, 28 Aug. 1988, 26; Wolf, *The Beauty Myth*, 231-232.

4. Findlay, "Buying the Perfect Body," 68-69.

5. Susan L. Wampler, citing the "Facial Plastic and Reconstructive Survey Study" in "Mirror: The Changing Face of Beauty," *Indianapolis Business Journal*, 19 Feb. 1990, III, 28.

6. Lisa M. Krieger, "New Face of Plastic Surgery," *San Francisco Examiner*, 1 Jan. 1989, A1; Naomi Wolf, "The Beauty Myth, Part Two: Under the Knife," *The Sunday Times*, 16 Sept. 1990, Sect. 7, 1; press kit from the American Society of Plastic and Reconstructive Surgeons Inc. and its Plastic Surgery Education Foundation; Susan Faludi, *Backlash: The Undeclared War Against American Women* (New York: Crown Publishing Group, 1991), 217. One statement released by the ASPRS stated: "There is a body of information that these deformities [small breasts] are really a disease." If not surgically corrected, the society even claimed that being flat-chested results in "a total lack of well-being."

7. *The New York Times Magazine*, 17 Apr. 1988, 57; Los Angeles Magazine, Feb. 1989; Teri Agins, "Boom in Busts," *The San Francisco Examiner*, 15 Dec. 1988, D1; "Go Curvy!: The Right Inches/The Right Places," *Mademoiselle*, Jan. 1988, 108; Wendy Kaminer, "Of Face Lifts and Feminism," *The New York Times*, 6 Sept. 1988, A23. (Sources for this paragraph from Faludi, *Backlash*, 216-217).

8. Findlay, "Buying the Perfect Body," 71.

9. "The Price of Beauty," *The Economist,* 11 Jan. 1992.

10. Rosen, "On the Cutting Edge," 60-70. Note: If you want to be like the men of Issachar and better understand the times we're living in—as the Bible mentions in 1 Chronicles 12:32—*People Weekly* provides plenty of clues.

11. Rosen, "On the Cutting Edge," 68.

12. Rosen, "On the Cutting Edge," 61.

13. U.S. House of Representatives Small Business Subcommittee, Spring 1989. See Federal Trade Commission Report, *Unqualified Doctors Performing Cosmetic Surgery: Policies and Enforcement Activities of the Federal Trade Commission,* Parts I, II, and III, serial no. 101-7.

14. Cable News Network, 19 Apr. 1989.

15. Findlay, "Buying the Perfect Body," 72; John Camp, *Plastic Surgery: The Kindest Cut* (New York: Henry Holt, 1989), 133-135; Freedman, *Beauty Bound,* 213; Elizabeth Morgan, *The Complete Book of Cosmetic Surgery* (New York: Warner Books, 1988), 119.

16. Camp, *Plastic Surgery,* 133.

17. Morgan, *The Complete Book of Plastic Surgery,* 117.

18. Morgan, *The Complete Book of Plastic Surgery,* 119.

19. Camp, *Plastic Surgery,* 132.

20. Rosen, "On the Cutting Edge," 61.

21. Karen Thomas, "Implants Leave Jones Scared, Mad," *USA Today,* 25 Feb. 1992, 6D.

22. Thomas, "Implants Leave Jones Scared, Mad," 6D.

23. Findlay, "Buying the Perfect Body," 75.

24. Philip J. Hilts, "FDA Seeks Halt in Breast Implants Made of Silicone; Cites Concern on Safety; Shift Comes After Devices' use in 2 Million U.S. Women Over Last 3 Decades," *The New York Times,* 7 Jan. 1992, A1; Editorial, "Wise Timeout on Breast Implants," *The New York Times,* 8 Jan. 1992, A16.

25 Philip J. Hilts, "Biggest Maker of Breast Implants Is Said to Be Abandoning Market," *The New York Times*, 19 Mar. 1992, A1; D'Arcy Jenish, "Dow Corning's Retreat," *Maclean's*, 30 Mar. 1992, 39.

26. Tim Smart, "Breast Implants: What Did the Industry Know, and When?" *Business Week*, 10 June 1991, 94-98; Jean Seligmann, "The Hazards of Silicone," *Newsweek*, 29 Apr. 1991, 56. The FDA didn't begin regulating medical devices until 1976: anything on the market before that time was "grandfathered in" and was assumed to be safe unless proven otherwise. In 1982, the FDA reclassified implants as potentially risky, but it wasn't until 1988 that they were placed in a category which required proof of their safety. In 1991 the FDA issued a 90-day warning to implant makers to prove their products safe—or take them off the market.

27. Arlene Fischer, "A Body to Die For," *Redbook Magazine*, Sept. 1991, 96.

28. Fischer, "A Body to Die For," 98.

29. Jean Seligmann, "The Hazards of Silicone," 56.

30. Philip J. Hilts, "FDA Restricts Use of Implants Pending Studies," *The New York Times*, 17 Apr. 1992, A1; Marian Segal, "Silicone Breast Implants: Available Under Tight Controls," *FDA Consumer*, June 1992, 6-10.

31. It has been estimated plastic surgeons' profits from doing 200,000 to 1,000,000 breast implant operations in the last 10 years alone has been between $168 and $374 million. These surgeries are not officially tallied by the U.S. Center for Health Statistics, so the exact number is not known; however, the FDA is assuming that about 150,000 women annually have undergone the procedure in recent years. (Jeff Nesmith, "Women May Be Warned of Implants," *The Atlanta Journal/The Atlanta Constitution*, 26 Sept. 1991, E7.) See also: Jeremy Weir, "Breast Frenzy," *Self*, April 1989.

32. Laura Shapiro, "What Is It with Women and Breasts?" *Newsweek*, 20 Jan. 1992, 57.

33. Fauldi, *Backlash*, 222. According to the ASPRS, the number of

plastic surgery procedures performed for breast reconstruction and to restore burn victims' appearance fell substantially in the late 1980s. Between 1984 and 1986, the number of breast reconstruction procedures fell from 98,000 to 57,200, and the number of burn reconstruction operations dipped from 23,200 to 20,400.

34. Faludi, *Backlash*, 214.

35. Ecclesiasticus 38:6-8, New English Bible, from the Apocrypha.

36. The Oath of Hippocrates, sixth century B.C.

37. The Oath of Asaph, sixth century A.D., written by Asaph Judaeus, a Hebrew physician. Note: both the Oath of Hippocrates and the Oath of Asaph also prohibited physicians from practicing abortion in any form.

38. Immanuel Jakobvits, *Jewish Bioethics*, quoted by Daniel Overduin and John Fleming, *Life in a Test-Tube*, (Adelaide, South Australia: Lutheran Publishing House, 1982), 192.

39. Overduin and Fleming, *Life in a Test-Tube*, 3.

40. See; "Scalpel Slaves Just Can't Quit!" *Newsweek*, 11 Jan. 1988 for more information on plastic surgery addiction. It states that for some women, "Neither cost, pain nor spectacular bruising [lessen] the desire for a little more whittling." In his survey of the patients of more than 300 plastic surgeons, psychiatrist Dr. Norman J. Knorr and his colleagues found that "insatiable" cosmetic surgery clients tend to have low self-esteem and intense feelings of inadequacy in their personal, sexual, and work relationships—characteristics common in other types of addicts as well. See also: Annette C. Hamburger, "Beauty Quest," *Psychology Today*, May 1988, 31. Yet most plastic surgeons lack adequate training to screen patients for potential surgical addiction.

Chapter 6

1. M. Solomon, ed., *The Psychology of Fashion* (Lexington, MA: Lexington Books, 1985).

2. "Fashion Fax: What Will Make You Buy?" *Glamour*, July 1992, 116.

3. Barbara Rudolph, "Beauty and the Bucks," *Time*, 7 Oct. 1991, 38.

4. "The Models: Their Lives, Loves and Money," *First For Women*, 27 Apr. 1992, 16.

5. Tom Fennell, "The Best in the World," *Maclean's*, 9 Dec. 1991, 37.

6. Fennell, "The Best in the World," 37.

7. Rick Tetzell, "Recession-Proof Supermodels," *Fortune*, 23 Mar.1992, 12.

8. Matt Rees, "Corporate America's Most Powerful People," *Forbes*, 26 May 1992, 164.

9. Rees, "Corporate America's Most Powerful People," 164.

10. The epitome of the sixties bustless, hipless look, Twiggy actually measured 31-22-32 in her heyday, though she's larger than that now.

11. *Orange County Register*, "Girlish Ideal Worries Some Health Experts," in *The Atlanta Journal/The Atlanta Constitution*, 19 May 1993, B5. See also: Rona Berg, "The Waif Farers," *The New York Times Magazine*, 21 Mar. 1993, 44-40.

12. "Girlish Ideals," *Orange County Register*, B5.

13. Mary Talbot, "Showing Too Much Too Soon," *Time*, 26 Apr. 1993, 59.

14. Talbot, "Showing Too Much," 59.

15. Linda Castrone and Rebecca Jones, "Traditional Women's Magazines Taking on a Sexier, Cosmo Tone," *The Atlanta Journal*, 15 May 1992, D2. When it comes to creating and marketing new magazines, sex is a big seller: of 679 magazines launched in 1992, 97 focused on sex. Runners-up were lifestyle (60), sports (40), and crafts, games, and hobbies (35). Source: *Samir Husni's Guide to New Consumer Magazines*, 1993, quoted in "USA Snapshots," *USA Today*, 24 May 1993, 1D.

16. Jeffry Scott, "Selling with Sexism," *The Atlanta Journal/ The Atlanta Constitution*, 24 Nov. 1991, H1.

17. Scott, "Selling with Sexism," H6.

18. Scott, "Selling with Sexism," H6.

19. Woody Hochswender, "Vogue Beauty: Appearance at Work," *Vogue*, Oct. 1991, 232,238.

20. "What Price Beauty?" *Glamour*, 302.

21. Hochswender, "Vogue Beauty," 230-231.

22. For women building a wardrobe on a budget, it's an expensive proposition—regardless of whether a classic look or trendier style is chosen: in a recent survey conducted by *Working Woman* magazine, 62 percent of respondents say they spend an average of $100-$300 on each outfit they wear to work. Source: Marcy E. Mullins, "The Cost of an Outfit at Work," *USA Today*, 11 Sept. 1992, 1D.

23. *People Weekly*, "The Little Princess," 22 June 1992, 96.

24. Matthew 6:25,28.

25. Matthew 6:29.

26. Kris Worrell, "The Interview Suit," *The Atlanta Journal/The Atlanta Constitution*, 16 May 1993, L6.

Chapter 7

1.   According to beauty historian Arthur Markham, "In the traditional view—and elements of the traditional view persisted well into the twentieth century—the major status characteristics were wealth and social position; beauty, apart from being an enticement to the sin of lust, was seen as a menace to both of these. In the 1960s beauty was universally praised and sought after; it had achieved a kind of parity with wealth and status, and certainly was no enemy of either." Marwick, *Beauty in History*, 343. See also: M. Webster and J. E. Driskell, "Beauty as Status," *American Journal of Sociology* (89) 1983: 140-165.

2.   Philippians 1:6.

3.   Psalm 103:13-16. See also Proverbs 31:30 and Ecclesiastes 1:14; Isaiah 28:4 and 40:6-8; 1 Peter 1:24.

4. Genesis 1:31; Psalm 19:1; Ecclesiastes 3:11; Romans 1:20.

5. 2 Samual 11:2 and Proverbs 6:25.

6. Synnott, "Truth and Goodness, Mirrors and Masks," 611.

7. Synnott, "Truth and Goodness, Mirrors and Masks," 611.

8. Genesis 6:1-8.

9 Arthur Marwick further explains why: "Beauty is that entirely physical phenomenon which has a profound effect on other people. . . The beautiful are those who are immediately sexually exciting to almost all members of the opposite sex (and sometimes to members of their own sex, as well). . . . We like to associate with a beautiful person; naturally if we have a chance, we like to go to bed with a beautiful person." (Marwick, *Beauty in History*, 44, 41.) For additional study, read: Marshall Dermer and Darrel L. Thiel, "When Beauty May Fail," *Journal of Personality and Social Psychology* 31 (1975), 1168-1176.

10. Genesis 12:11-12.

11. Genesis 12:18-19.

12. Genesis 20:1-18.

13. Genesis 26:1-11.

14. 2 Samuel 11:2-4.

15. 2 Samuel 11:6-12:23.

16. Genesis 27:1-29.

17. Genesis 31:19-35.

18. Esther 4:1.

19. Esther 4:13-14.

20. Esther 9:18-20.

21. *The Random House College Dictionary*, rev., s.v. "gorgeous."

22. *The Random House College Dictionary*, rev., s.v. "adornment."

23. 2 Corinthians 3:18.

24. 1 Peter 3:3-4, NEB, (emphasis added).

Chapter 8

- C. S. Lewis, "The Weight of Glory," in *The Weight of Glory* (Grand Rapids, MI: Eerdmans, 1975):14-15.

1. A. G. Miller, "Role of Physical Attractiveness in Impression Formation," *Psychonomic Science* (19) 1970: 241-243; J. F. Cross and J. Cross, "Age, Sex, Race and the Perception of Facial Beauty," *Developmental Psychology* (5) 1971: 437-442; K. K. Dion, E. Berscheid, and E. Walster, "What Is Beautiful Is Good," 285-290; E. Berscheid and E. Walster, "Physical Attractiveness," *Advances in Experimental Social Psychology*, vol. 7, L. Berkowitz, ed. (New York: Academic Press, 1974); John Liggett, *The Human Face* (New York: Stein and Day, 1974); M. K. Hill and H. A. Lando, "Physical Attractiveness and Sex-Role Stereotypes in Impression Formation." *Perceptual and Motor Skills* 47 (1976): 1251-1255; G. R. Adams, "Physical Attractiveness Research: Toward a Developmental Social Psychology of Beauty," *Human Development* 20 (1977): 217-239; T. F. Cash, "Physical Attractiveness: An Annotated Bibliography of Theory and Research in the Behavioral Sciences," *JSAS Catalog of Selected Documents in Psychology* 11 (1981): 85 (Ms. No. 2370); G. L. Patzer, *The Physical Attractiveness Phenomena* (New York: Plenum Press, 1985); T. A. Brown, T. F. Cash, and S. W. Noles, "Perceptions of Physical Attractiveness Among College Students: Selected Determinant and Methodological Matters," *Journal of Social Psychology* 126 (1986): 305-316; Bruce Bower, "Average Attractions: Scientists Break Down the Essence of Physical Beauty," *Science News* 137 (1990): 298; Constance Holden, "Ordinary Is Beautiful: What Makes Faces Attractive," *Science* 248 (1990): 306; Judith H. Langlois, Lori A. Roggman, and Loretta A. Rieser-Danner, "Infants' Differential Social Responses to Attractive and Unattractive Faces," *Developmental Psychology* 26 (1990),153-157; A. H. Eagly et al.,"What Is Beautiful Is Good, But . . : A Meta-Analytic Review of Research on the Physical Attractiveness Stereotype," *Psychological Bulletin* 110 (1991): 109-128; Judith H. Langlois et al., "Facial Diversity and Infant Preferences for Attractive Faces," *Developmental Psychology* 27 (1991): 79-86.

2. Ezekiel 36:26.

3. Paul Brand and Philip Yancey, *In His Image* (Grand Rapids, MI: Zondervan, 1984), 40, 42, 46. For additional study on the image of Christ, see: 2 Corinthians 4:4-18 and Colossians 1: 15-27, 3:10.

4. C. S. Lewis, *That Hideous Strength* (New York: Macmillan Publishing Company, 1946, 1965), 317-319. Used by permission, copyright: The Bodley Head, London England.

5. Acts 17:28.

6. Romans 12:1-2, NEB.

7. Dick Keyes, *Beyond Identity* (Ann Arbor, MI: Servant Books, 1984), 102-103, 106-107; feminine pronouns added.

8. Keyes, *Beyond Identity*, 99.

9. Colossians 1:27, NEB.

Chapter 9

- Charles Kingsley, quoted in *The Oxford Book of Prayer*, George Appleton (Ed.) (Oxford: Oxford University Press, 1985), 121.

- Roger Steer ed., *The George Muller Treasury* (Wheaton, IL: Crossway Books, 1987), 26.

1. Michael Crichton, *Jurassic Park* (New York: Alfred A. Knopf, Inc., 1990), 12-13.

2. One definition of the word idol—another word used to describe a false god—is "any person or thing devotedly or excessively admired" (*The Random House College Dictionary*, rev.).

3. 1 Corinthians 10:23-33.

4. Hebrews 13:5, NEB.

5. Acts 17:21.

6. Matthew 4:10, AMP.

7. For further study, see: 1 Corinthians 10:1-14; Psalm 115:4-8; Psalm 135:15-18; Galatians 5:16-6:10; Ephesians 5:1-10; Colossians

3:5-17; 1 Peter 4:1-11; 1 John 5:21; and Psalm 97:7.

8. Matthew 6:33a NKJV.

9. R. C. Sproul, *Pleasing God* (Wheaton, IL: Tyndale, 1988), 31-32.

10. 2 Corinthians 10:5, AMP.

11. Matthew 6:24; James 1:2-8.

12. George MacDonald, *Unspoken Sermons*, 2nd series, "Self-denial," 1855, in C. S. Lewis, *George MacDonald: An Anthology* (New York: Macmillan Publishing Company, 1947), 68.

13. Matthew 10:39, AMP.

14. Matthew 22:37-39.

15. Arlene Dahl, *Always Ask a Man: Arlene Dahl's Key to Femininity* (Englewood Cliffs, NJ: Prentice-Hall, 1965), 5.

16. 1 Timothy 2:8-9.

17. Ephesians 6:14-17; Colossians 3:12-13.

18. Galatians 5:22-23.

19. James 1:5, 3:13-18.

20. Matthew. 7:7-11

Chapter 10

Phillips Brooks, quoted by Gladys Hunt in *Ms. Means Myself* (Grand Rapids, MI: Zondervan, 1972), 17.

1. Oswald Chambers, *My Utmost for His Highest* (New York: Dodd, Mead & Co., 1935), 89.

2. Matthew 18:2-4.

3. John White, *Changing on the Inside* (Ann Arbor, MI: Vine Books, 1991): 229-230 (emphasis added).

4. Isaiah 40:31. See also Psalm 103:5.

5. Philippians 3:14 (emphasis added).

6. White, *Changing on the Inside*, 230.

7. In his Epistle to the Romans, the Apostle Paul expresses the problem this way: "They exchanged the truth of God for a lie and worshiped and served created things rather than the Creator— who is forever praised. Amen" (Romans 1:25).

8. Eugene H. Peterson, *A Long Obedience in the Same Direction: Discipleship in an Instant Society* (Downer's Grove, IL: InterVarsity Press, 1980), 21.

9. Peterson, *A Long Obedience,* 23 (emphasis added).

10 Peterson, *A Long Obedience,* 25-26, 29 (emphasis added).

11. To see these pictures of femininity drawn from the Bible, read: 2 Corinthians 3:18 (in relationship to Jesus, we are *all* feminine as the Bride of Christ reflects the glory of God); Psalm 17:7-9 and Psalm 91:4 (female birds—not male—typically shelter their young under their wings); Isaiah 40:11 (God gathers the weak to His bosom); Isaiah 66:10-13 (comforting and provision); Luke 13:34 (Jesus compares Himself to a mother hen); Proverbs 3:13-18 (wisdom portrayed as a woman rather than as a man); Jeremiah 31:15-17 (Rachel weeping for Israel's defenseless children); Song of Songs 4:16-5:1 (descriptions of the interplay between masculine/lover and feminine/beloved); Proverbs 31:10-31 (creativity, provision of shelter, and industry); and Exodus 1:15-21 (midwives rescuing Hebrew children from death). In addition, throughout nature God has designated the female animal or part of a plant to be the fruit-bearer, and the male the seed-sower.

12. St. John Chrysostom, "The True Adornment of Woman," The First Instruction, article 34, *Baptismal Instructions* (Westminster, MD: The Newman Press), 36-37.

13. Chrysostom, "The True Adornment," article 35,37.

14. Chrysostom, "The True Adornment," article 37, 38.

15. Chrysostom, "The True Adornment," article 38, 39.

16. Chrysostom, "The True Adornment of Woman," articles 42, 43, 185-186.

17. Chrysostom, "The True Adornment of Woman," article 46, 187.

18. Chrysostom, "The True Adornment of Woman," article 47, 187.

19. Lewis, *George MacDonald: An Anthology*, 69.

20. 1 Peter 3:4, J. B. Phillips

21. Hannah More, "Self-Love," in Sherwood Eliot Wirt, ed., *Spiritual Awakening* (Wheaton, IL: Crossway Books, 1986), 76.

22. More, *"Self-Love,"* p. 74.

23. John White, *Flirting With the World* (Downer's Grove, IL: InterVarsity Press, 1982),99,102 (emphasis added). The Sermon on the Mount (Matthew 5:1-7:28; Luke 6:17-46) is worth reading regularly as an encouragement to keep seeking the Kingdom of Heaven first. Other good passages to consider frequently include: 1 Peter 1:13-2:3; Ephesians 4:22-24, 5:1-2; 1 Timothy 6:6-19; Colossians 3:1-4; Colossians 3:5-17; Philippians 4:6-9; 1 John 2:15-17; 2 Corinthians 10: 3-5; Galatians 5:16-26; Romans 12:1-3; Hebrews 12:1-12; and Titus 2:11-14.

24. 1 Corinthians 6:19-20

25. Matthew 10:16.